DEDICATION
To my mother and father:
For never believing type 1 diabetes would hold me back.
Thank you for supporting me in everything I do.

HIGHS & LOWS
of TYPE 1 DIABETES

THE ULTIMATE GUIDE
FOR TEENS AND YOUNG ADULTS

VALUABLE TIPS, TRICKS, AND ADVICE FROM
A VETERAN YOUNG ADULT WITH TYPE 1 DIABETES

PATRICK McALLISTER

FOREWORD BY STUART A. WEINZIMER, MD

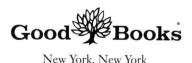

Good Books

New York, New York

Good Books books may be purchased in bulk at special discounts
for sales promotion, corporate gifts, fund-raising, or educational
purposes. Special editions can also be created to specifications.
For details, contact the Special Sales Department, Good Books,
307 West 36th Street, 11th Floor, New York, NY 10018 or info@
skyhorsepublishing.com.

Good Books in an imprint of Skyhorse Publishing, Inc.®, a Delaware
corporation.

Visit our website at www.goodbooks.com.

10 9 8 7 6 5 4 3 2 1

Library of Congress Cataloging-in-Publication Data is available on file.

Cover design by Jenny Zemanek
Cover photo credit iStockphoto

Print ISBN: 978-1-68099-298-4
Ebook ISBN: 978-1-68099-299-1

Printed in China

CONTENTS

FOREWORD

The day I met Patrick was just an ordinary work day for me, but it was not an ordinary day for him. It will forever be one of the most significant days of his life: the day he was diagnosed with type 1 diabetes. It is often said that while we can't control which challenges we may face in life, we can control how we respond to these challenges. And from that very first day, Patrick has met the challenges of diabetes head-on. Diabetes is unusual among many chronic illnesses in the way that it pervades *everything* in a person's life. It affects every aspect of one's daily routine and makes itself present at the grandest moments and the most mundane. Managing life with diabetes is not just about remembering to take your medicine; it is about learning how to navigate every aspect of life with a new, unwelcome partner.

Success with diabetes requires resilience, support, and a good sense of humor, all of which can be found in Patrick's book, which explains in a direct, straightforward, unvarnished manner what a teen or young adult needs to understand about diabetes to succeed. *Highs & Lows of Type 1 Diabetes* speaks directly to the teen about such important and sometimes difficult topics, such as coping with the diagnosis, learning how to tell friends, and juggling diabetes with sex, drugs, and alcohol—all in an honest, relatable, nonjudgmental approach. Teens and young adults will find in this book the information and advice needed to learn about their illness, gain control over it, and deal with those tough days when diabetes gets the better of them—from a person who has "been there."

Ten years ago, the summer Patrick was diagnosed with diabetes was also the summer that we published our first study on the "artificial pancreas," an automated insulin delivery system that promised to improve the health and quality of life of people living with type 1 diabetes. Today, as Patrick's book is published, the first generation of these systems is now available. And in the next ten years, further discovery will undoubtedly continue to ease the burden of diabetes. But as Patrick reminds us, whatever technological or pharmacological advancements arrive on the scene, the most important tools to manage living with diabetes will always be learning as much as you can, finding support in friends and family, and meeting the challenges head-on with resilience, humor, and grace.

Stuart A. Weinzimer, MD
Professor of Pediatrics
Yale University School of Medicine
September 28, 2017

INTRODUCTION

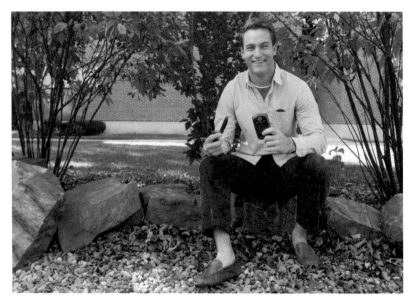

Patrick McAllister. © Sam Prue

What is diabetes?

Diabetes is a disease that affects how your body uses food and sugar. An organ called the **pancreas** makes a chemical called **insulin**, which is a molecular key. Insulin unlocks your cells, allowing sugar to enter and be turned into energy. We need energy to do all the things we love to do: play soccer, hang out with friends, and ace that really difficult math test. Diabetes is a disease in which your body has trouble making insulin (the key) and so no cells can be unlocked. Without the key, you cannot get any energy.

There are two main types of diabetes. The most common is **type 2 diabetes** (T2D). This type of diabetes is commonly a result of poor diet over a long period of time, but it also has a strong genetic component. Eventually, a poor diet puts so much pressure on your pancreas that it stops responding and cannot do its job. As a result, your body becomes resistant to the insulin you are producing. Because your body essentially views your insulin as the "wrong key," your cells cannot be unlocked. Some people with T2D require daily insulin injections, but with good diet and exercise, many people with T2D are completely insulin free.

Type 1 diabetes (T1D), on the other hand, is when your body simply stops producing the key altogether. Your body actually attacks the cells in your pancreas that make insulin. These cells are called β-**cells**, and once damaged, they stop producing insulin. And as we know, without a key, you cannot unlock anything. T1D is normally diagnosed during childhood, but it is not uncommon to see people diagnosed as late as in their twenties. I was diagnosed with T1D when I was twelve years old.

So how did I get T1D? Most likely, T1D is a result of both your **genes** and the environment around you. On the genetic side, one or both of your parents probably gave you one or more genes associated with T1D. You might even be able to figure out where the gene(s) came from by looking at your family and seeing if anyone else has T1D. In my family, my cousin on my mother's side of the family has T1D, so I assume my mom may have given me one or more genes associated with the disease. Even though this is good knowledge to have, just remember that your parents did not give you T1D on purpose. It happened by chance, so do not hang this over their heads, saying, "It's your fault I have this." It is nobody's fault. Unfortunately, we do not yet completely know what genes are associated with T1D, so we cannot prevent people from getting it.

As stated earlier, T1D is not solely genetic. The environment also plays a critical role in this equation. The best example I can provide is to consider T1D in identical twins. Interestingly, even though twins have the exact same DNA, there are instances in which only one of them gets T1D. Weird, right? Like our incomplete knowledge of genes and T1D, we are not yet sure what external factors cause the disease either.

At this point, T1D may seem like a complete mystery. We do not know what genes cause it, and we do not know what environmental factors cause it. *Great!* So, what do we know? Well, we actually know quite a bit. We know how to control it and how to make it manageable in everyday life. When you think of the daunting diagnosis of "type 1 diabetes," do not imagine it as a scary disease that is going to ruin your life. T1D is *not* a death sentence at all; it's just a lifestyle change. Millions of people around the world manage life with T1D and go on to be very successful and happy people. Jay Cutler is a quarterback in the NFL; Halle Berry is a successful actress; Nick Jonas is a famous singer; and Sonia Sotomayor is a Supreme Court judge. Not bad!

Sure, T1D is a struggle at times, but if you can learn to control it, there is nothing stopping you from reaching your goals. In fact, you may find that T1D helps you in certain parts of your life. For example, people with T1D are generally more prepared for life because it gives them a sense of responsibility, independence, and discipline. I am not trying to twist this around and say that T1D is a good thing. It stinks, and sometimes you just want to scream it from the rooftops. But it is manageable; you just have to stick with it. And it does have its perks.

This book is meant to help guide you through the everyday challenges we face with T1D. From getting diagnosed in the hospital to leaving for college, I am going to tackle every scenario in between with the hope that you can find some of my tips and experiences helpful. Having said that, know that you don't have to read this entire book at once and memorize every line. Take it one chapter at a time. Also, read the sections that are going to be most helpful to you. For example, you don't have to read the section on college (yet) if you are in the seventh grade.

Another important note is to read this book with an open mind. Put more plainly, do not take the contents of this book as the absolute truth. I write from my own experiences and the experiences of other people with T1D who I know personally. If you find that something you do is successful for you and differs from what I say, that's okay. In fact, an essential key to T1D management is understanding that T1D is different for everyone. Your body acts differently than my body and Nick Jonas's body. While many things are similar, some things are different. The one person who knows your T1D best is you—not your doctors, not your parents, not your friends—*you*. Listen to your body, and take what you can from my tips and experiences.

Patrick McAllister

1

DIAGNOSIS AND THOSE
FIRST FEW WEEKS

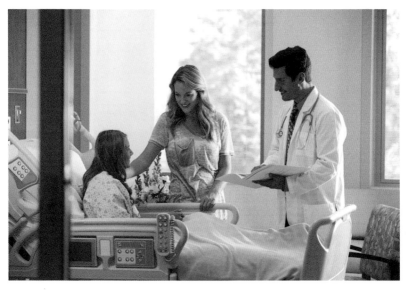

The best way I can give advice in this first chapter is to tell you the
story of my diagnosis. I always enjoy hearing other diagnosis stories
and comparing them to my own, and maybe you do too. It is odd
how similar diagnosis stories can be, despite differing dates and

locations. As I describe my experiences, I will pause and provide some helpful tips along the way.

I was diagnosed with T1D when I was twelve years old. It happened toward the end of the summer before I was about to enter the seventh grade. I went to my doctor's office on August 11 for a routine checkup as it was getting close to my thirteenth birthday. Before we left for the doctor's, I remember playing soccer with my younger sister outside in my front yard. To be honest, I was not even thinking about the doctor's office; my mind was on the delicious ice cream I was going to get after the short and painless visit. There was a McDonald's located right across from the doctor's office, and after every checkup, my mom would treat me and my sister to a McDonald's ice cream. My favorite was the M&M McFlurry.

We got to the office in the late morning. My doctor went through all the tests and yearly booster shots, and when he came back into our waiting room, he had a troubled look on his face. He told us that when they tested my urine, they found an unusually high amount of sugar. I had no idea what he was talking about, so I looked over at my mom to see her reaction. She remained very calm, even when the doctor told us we might need to go to the hospital. He said he would call us in a couple of hours, and we left the doctor's office in silence. After the appointment, we skipped our McFlurry tradition, at which point I knew the situation was worse than I had originally thought.

We headed home and waited in anticipation. My mom started to break down and cry a little, which made me really nervous. She told me I might have T1D, at which point my mind jumped immediately to my friend Jonah. Jonah was diagnosed with T1D when he was very young, and I remember hearing stories of his struggles. I particularly remembered him telling me about the multitude of test strips that littered his house. I always joked with him about this, but now it no longer seemed so funny. The thought of the "test strip clutter" overwhelmed me, and I immediately started to cry.

"Mom, I don't want diabetes. I don't want test strips all over the house. I want our house to stay clean." Looking back, it is kind of funny that out of all the things I could have been worried about regarding T1D, I chose to become completely terrified by the possibility of a few test strips lying on the floor. My mom tried to comfort me, but I was past that. I was panicking.

TIP: Here is the first of many tips I will share with you throughout this chapter: *Do not* panic. It is a natural response to lose control temporarily when you get bad news like this, but try to stay as calm as possible. It is not the end of the world. I know how stressful this kind of situation can be, but if you stay calm, the entire process will go much smoother. Take some deep breaths, assess your situation, and then evaluate what you can do to make it better.

We got the call from my doctor after a couple of hours. He told us to go to the hospital. We packed some changes of clothes, dropped my little sister off at my aunt's house, and headed up to Yale New Haven Hospital in Connecticut. When we arrived, I started to panic once again. I do not care what age you are; hospitals are crazy places. There are always people running around, machines beeping, and patients yelling; it's a zoo!

My parents checked us in, and we were put in a small waiting room. Not too long after, a nurse came in and checked my blood sugar: 488. I did not know what this number meant at the time, but I assumed it was not good news because we were immediately relocated to another hospital room. This was all so odd to me. *What's the big deal? I feel fine.* The nurse explained that the children's diabetes wing of the hospital was full, so they had to temporarily admit me on the general floor. In the room, they hooked me up to an IV and started treating me with insulin. I had no idea what any of this stuff was, but that was soon about to change.

There is not really anything you can do when sitting in a hospital bed except read a book or watch TV. I chose the latter. My mom had never let me watch *Family Guy*, but when it came on the channel, she did not say anything (it's safe to say I took advantage of the situation). We sat and watched *Family Guy* for an hour or so, before a nurse came in to check my blood sugar again. He explained that he needed to do this to see if my blood sugar level was getting better. He asked if he could draw blood from one of my fingers. It did not hurt that much, but it was not comfortable, either. He inserted a small, flat stick into a handheld machine that drew up the blood on my finger. The little machine in his hand beeped twice, and then he smiled, saying that my sugars were looking better. That reassurance gave my parents and me some short-lived comfort.

After another hour passed, a doctor came into the room with a bunch of college-age young adults with white lab coats and clipboards. He seemed nice—average height, short brown hair, glasses, and a big smile across his face. His lab coat read *Dr. Stuart Weinzimer*.

"How are you today, Patrick? My name is Dr. Weinzimer. I am going to be one of your diabetes doctors. These are some students of mine. Do you mind if they stay and watch?" I shook my head without saying a word. Just another overwhelming factor about this hospital: seven bright-white lab coats standing in your room, scrutinizing you like you are some kind of new discovery. He started by asking me some light questions, like what grade I was in and what sports I played, probably to try to ease some of my nerves. Then he started with the real information. He began to explain to me what T1D was, using the "key" analogy. He also went through the basics of what different terms meant, such as *blood sugar* and *insulin*. I tried to take in as much information as I could, but a lot of it just went straight over my head. After he finished, he asked if I had any questions; I immediately shook my head "no." I was not thinking of questions at that time, and even if I had one, I was too scared to ask.

TIP: It is okay to ask questions; in fact, it is actually a good idea. I wish someone had told me this before I entered the hospital; it would have totally changed my approach while I was there. You don't have to force a question out of your mouth for the sake of asking, but if you *do* have a question or a topic you do not understand, get clarification. No question is too dumb. This sounds so simple, and I bet most people will look at this tip and say, "Duh, of course. I always ask questions if I have them. Why wouldn't I?" But I can guarantee you that most of us would remain as silent as I did when put in the same situation. Be bold. The more you ask, the more the doctors and nurses can help you; it is what they're there for. And while they are very smart, they are not mind readers. Trust them, and trust yourself.

Before leaving my room, Dr. Weinzimer patted me on the shoulder, saying, "Everything is going to be okay." I wish I had been able to see the truth in that statement at the time, instead of shrugging it off as something doctors say because they are supposed to.

When suppertime rolled around, my nurse came in with a dinner menu. I knew what I wanted the second I saw it: *pizza*. I love pizza! Have you ever gotten that dumb question, *If you were stranded on an island and could only eat one thing for the rest of your life, what would it be?* Well, my answer was, is, and always will be cheese pizza. Upon closer examination, I noticed the number "101" printed next to the words "Personal Pizza." I asked what it meant. The nurse explained that this referred to the number of carbohydrates in the meal and added that I could only have between seventy and ninety carbs in a meal, at which point I immediately sank back into my bed. The staff must have taken pity on me, because they said they would make an exception. When my food finally arrived some forty-five minutes later, I was starving. It was a puny little pizza, probably meant for an eight-year-old, and the crust did not look particularly appetizing—but I did not care. All I wanted to do was sink my teeth into that molten cheese and bright-red sauce. However, before I could eat anything, the nurse said that he had to give me a shot in my arm so I *could* eat. He took out a needle and drew up some clear liquid from a vial.

"What's that?" I asked the nurse.

"It's insulin. It's going to allow you to eat." He took the needle with the insulin in it and punctured the tip into the side of my arm. I am not going to lie; it hurt. He pushed the insulin in and then pulled the needle out.

"So I have to do that every time before I eat?" I asked.

"Yup. That wasn't so bad, was it?" the nurse replied.

What are you talking about?! That was terrible, I thought. It took me a minute to get over the fact that I was going to have to inject myself every time I wanted to eat for the rest of my life. When I finally took the first bite out of my pizza, I realized I was not that hungry anymore. For the rest of the night, doctors and nurses filtered in and out of my room, testing my blood sugar and checking my IV. I went to sleep discouraged; I felt beaten. I was consumed by this feeling that all the fun was over and that the rest of my life was going to be a living hell. Needless to say, I did not actually get much sleep that night.

The next morning, I ate a breakfast of two small boxes of Honey Nut Cheerios, along with the now routine finger prick and shot in the arm. Soon after, someone came in and said that a room had cleared up on the children's diabetes floor and that I was to be moved there shortly. Once I was situated in my new room, another doctor came in and greeted me. His name was Dr. William Tamborlane. He was much older than Dr. Weinzimer (you could tell by his shiny white hair and pudgy, wrinkly face), and a little heavier too; and when he smiled (which was always), his eyes squinted to the point where you could barely see them. He honestly looked like the happiest doctor in the entire hospital.

"Well, hello there, Patrick. How are we doing today?" he said in a big booming voice.

"Good," I timidly replied. I never understood why people say "good" when they are really anything but "good." We talked for a while, and he cracked a few good jokes, which made me feel a lot better. As it turned out, Dr. Tamborlane lived in the same town as me. We talked about where we lived and how I had ridden my bike past his house dozens of times on my way to our town beach. It was nice to talk to someone about something other than diabetes for a change. After he left, I felt motivated and a lot better about my situation; for the first time, it seemed like I could handle this "diabetes thing." I decided I was done being cooped up in that hospital bed. I just wanted to go home. I spoke with my parents and doctors and asked to have several of my appointments moved to earlier times. Those appointments included one with a doctor who showed me and my parents how to administer insulin shots and another with a nutritionist who taught me about carbohydrates.

When the "injection" doctor came into the room, I was nervous. I hated those big needles. But when he used my arm to demonstrate how to inject insulin, I could barely feel anything. I was so surprised! *How did the injection suddenly not hurt compared to the one I had received earlier?* It turned out that the only needles the nurses had access to when I was located on the general floor were generic needles, ones much bigger than the regular insulin needles people with T1D are accustomed to using. In fact, a regular insulin needle is much smaller. When it came time for my parents to try it, my mom decided to go first. She was a natural. She knew just the right amount of force to use to get the needle in without hurting me too much. My dad was a completely different story, however. When it was his turn, he took the syringe in his hand and lined up his shot, as if my arm was a dartboard. He drilled the needle into my arm.

"*Ouch!* What the heck was that, Dad?"

"Oops. I'm sorry, Pat. I didn't mean to hurt you." We joked about it after, and I told him I was just being a wimp, but I could tell that he felt bad about hurting me. Looking back, I regret not making more of an effort to reassure him that he had not done anything wrong.

TIP: Be kind to your parents throughout this affair. This whole diagnosis process is about you, but you are not the only one on this rollercoaster. Your parents are right there next to you, and, believe me, they feel terrible and helpless that they cannot do anything to help you. Over the years, my dad has said on countless occasions, "Patrick, if I could take your diabetes away and put it on myself, I would. I would do it in a heartbeat. You know that, right?" I have a feeling that all parents would say the same thing. They might not be the best at injecting you with insulin, and they might not understand everything that is going on with your T1D, but they care more about you than you could ever imagine. You might have to take some time to explain certain information to them if they are having trouble understanding. But trust me, you need them, and they need you. If you are fortunate enough to have supportive parents like I do, they will always be a sturdy rock you can lean on throughout your life, but every now and then you have to be that rock for them too. If you all can learn to be support systems for each other, the whole process will become tremendously easier.

And for those of you who might not have the most supportive parents in the world, do not worry. There will be other people in your life who will want to help you with your T1D—your siblings, friends, teachers, and doctors, just to name a few. Above all else, know that you are not alone.

My last appointment was with a nutritionist. At the time, I was very anxious because I knew I was so close to being able to return home to my own bed, but looking back, the nutritionist appointment was the most helpful meeting during my stay at the hospital. She taught me what carbohydrates are and what foods to look out for. We talked for well over an hour, even though it was only supposed to be a thirty-minute meeting, and before she left, she gave me a carb-counting book to bring home with me. I thought it was going to be useless, but I ended up using it quite a bit during the first month or two after returning home.

Finally, my nurse took the IV out of my arm. My parents signed some papers, and I was now ready to go home. Though I was supposed to stay in the hospital for four days and three nights, I ended up spending only two nights.

TIP: When you are learning all this new information (insulin, carbs, etc.), go at your own pace. If information is coming at you too fast, tell the doctors to slow down. On the other hand, if you are comfortable with everything you are learning, like I was, ask for the process to be sped up. If you choose to do this, however, just be careful of cramming everything into a short amount of time. These first couple of days can be overwhelming, but you need to learn as much as you can. Do not just fly through everything because you want to get through it and return home, only to realize later on that you cannot remember anything the doctors told you. Be smart and move through the hospital process at a pace that is comfortable for you.

We got home around seven in the evening. When we walked in through the front door, I was overcome by an incredible feeling. I looked around at the familiar spaces of my kitchen and the family room down the hall, and I realized I would never again be in this house without my diabetes. It was the first time I thought of it as "*my* diabetes." I had accepted it. It was mine, and I was going to manage it. I was not going to let this disease defeat me, despite everything I had been through in the past seventy-two hours. The next couple of days were a struggle. It was weird having to use a measuring cup to measure out cereal at breakfast and having to inject myself multiple times every day. But as time went on, it got easier. I fell into a routine of checking my blood sugar before every meal and taking my insulin. I got good with counting carbs too. Eventually, I grew confident in my ability to count carbs and stopped using the carb book. I knew, for instance, that a glass of milk is about fifteen carbs and three Oreos are about twenty-five carbs.

A few weeks after my diagnosis, my aunt, uncle, and three older cousins, who lived three hours away from us, visited for a few days to help us paint our kitchen. The oldest of my cousins, Casey, also had T1D, and that, coupled with the fact that our kitchen did not actually need painting, made it very clear why they had traveled down to "help" us. Casey was probably in college at the time and had been diagnosed as a kid too. I thought it was nice that they wanted to help, but the last thing I wanted was a "pity party" for me. I hate being pitied, especially if it comes from my own family; I just wanted to handle this thing on my own. But you know what? Having my cousin there for those couple of days was pretty awesome. She told me about her diagnosis story and how, unlike me, she had lost a ton of weight before she ended up in the hospital. She had been drinking and peeing nonstop for over a week before anyone realized something was wrong. It made me feel like my diagnosis experience was a walk in the park. She also gave me some tips on eating, such as what I should do if I am hungry but my routine does not allow for any more carbs (answer: a spoonful of peanut butter will do the trick). Her younger sister and brother were also very helpful. They talked with my sister about what it was like living with a sibling who has T1D, and they also shared some funny stories.

Once, Casey and my second oldest cousin, Anna, were walking together on a beach boardwalk when, suddenly, Casey started feeling a low blood sugar coming on. Casey sat down so she would not fall, and Anna started to panic. Anna told Casey to wait at the bench while she went off to find sugar to correct Casey's low blood sugar. Anna ran into the nearest pizza shop, screaming for someone to help and that she needed sugar for her sister who has T1D. A man from behind the counter asked if Coca-Cola would help, and Anna yelled back, "Are you crazy? That's not a Diet Coke! She can't have that! She has diabetes!" Anna proceeded to storm out of the pizza shop without getting anything for her sister (in fact, Coca-Cola in that instance would have been the perfect solution to get Casey's blood sugar levels up). My sister and I laughed throughout the entire story, especially when Anna told us about her "lapse of judgment." As someone with T1D, I always find it funny to hear about another person's own troubles with T1D (as long as the story ends on a good note). Perhaps it is because I am secretly relieved that I am not the only one going through these scenarios daily.

TIP: When people learn about your diagnosis, they might contact you and your parents to offer help. Do not be stubborn. Accept the help. I used to think I was accepting acts of pity, but I was wrong; you are simply accepting assistance and, more important, friendship. My aunt, uncle, and cousins knew they could help by simply showing up with smiles on their faces. Though I could have managed on my own, it was nice and comforting to chat with people who had been through the same hardships as me. My cousins made me and my sister laugh about the experiences they had gone through, and it was the first time I connected diabetes with anything funny. So, whenever someone offers help, do not hesitate or think, *they are only doing this because they feel bad for me.* Stop being stubborn and embrace the help in front of you. Not everyone is lucky enough to be offered this kind of help, and you never know how long it is going to last. Take advantage of it.

As time went on, I continued to learn new things about my T1D: how to successfully manage it and what to do in certain situations. I hope the rest of this book will prove helpful so you do not have to learn things the hard way, like I did. I had to go through a lot of trial and error in dealing with my T1D, and I hope I can eliminate some of that from your experience.

2

CARBOHYDRATES—HOW TO EAT AND DRINK WITH T1D

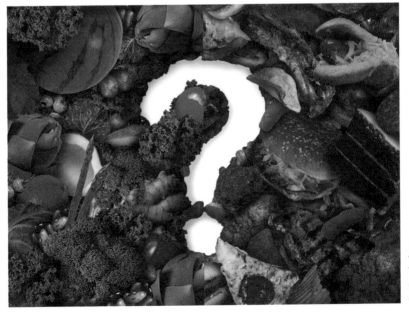

The part of life that undoubtedly changes the most when you are diagnosed with T1D is eating. I was diagnosed when I was twelve, and I am now twenty-one. And since I've managed to basically eat nonstop from ages thirteen to eighteen, I consider myself a true expert on eating with T1D. In this chapter, I will answer some basic questions about how to eat with T1D, as well as provide some tips on handling tricky food-related situations. Before I begin, a first piece of advice would be to get one of those little carbohydrate-counting books (like the one my nutritionist gave me at the hospital). It is a great tool. On top of providing nutritional information on regular foods, some of these books even include information about various fast food places and restaurants. If you are more technologically savvy than me, another option is to download one of the many nutritional applications on your smartphone. Those apps constantly update too, so you will always be kept in the loop with the newest changes in nutritional information. Eventually, you will be able to count carbs on your own, but until then, these tools are extremely helpful when you are first starting out.

WHAT ARE CARBOHYDRATES (CARBS)?

When I was diagnosed with T1D, one of the first things I had to wrap my mind around was **carbohydrates (carbs)**. What are they? How do they differ from sugar and calories? And why do I have to keep track of them?

First, let's get the basics down: carbohydrates are sugars. When you think about it, this makes complete sense. Water and meat do not have any sugar in them, and therefore do not have any carbs, while fruit and candy have tons of sugar and, likewise, tons of carbs. Generally, the sweeter the food, the more carbs it has. However, carbs also encompass starch, which is basically anything that would fit in the lowest part of the food pyramid—bread, cereal, pasta, rice, and so on (we will talk about the different kinds of carbs later).

The reason you have to count carbs is because carbs are the raw material your cells break down to turn into energy. Carbohydrates break down into glucose, and glucose is transformed into energy. Since people with T1D do not produce insulin (the key) that unlocks and opens cells to allow to glucose (carbs) inside, we must inject insulin into ourselves. The more carbs you eat, the more insulin is required to balance out those carbs. However, the amount of insulin people with T1D need for specific portions of food varies from person to person. For example, if two people with T1D eat a banana (about twenty-five carbs), one person might need to inject only one unit of insulin to cover those carbs, while the other person might need to inject two. You and your doctor will find out how your body responds to carbs within the first few weeks of your diagnosis.

HOW ARE "CARBS" DIFFERENT FROM "SUGARS" AND "CALORIES"?

Nutrition Facts

Serving Size 3 oz. (85g)
Serving Per Container 2

Amount Per Serving

Calories 200	Calories from Fat 120

% Daily Value*

Total Fat 15g	**20 %**
Saturated Fat 5g	**28 %**
Trans Fat 3g	
Cholesterol 30mg	**10 %**
Sodium 650mg	**28 %**
Total Carbohydrate 30g	**10 %**
Dietary Fiber 0g	**0 %**
Sugars 5g	
Protein 5g	

Vitamin A 5%	•	Vitamin C 2%
Calcium 15%	•	Iron 5%

*Percent Daily Values are based on a 2,000 calorie diet. Your Daily Values may be higher or lower depending on your calorie needs.

	Calories	2,000	2,500
Total Fat	Less than	65g	80g
Sat Fat	Less than	20g	25g
Cholesterol	Less than	300mg	300mg
Sodium	Less than	2,400mg	2,400mg
Total Carbonhydrate		300mg	375g
Dietary Fiber		25g	30g

Sugars are a type of carbohydrate. In fact, if you look at any nutritional facts label on the side of a food product, the "Sugars" tab is a sublabel underneath the "Total Carbohydrate" tab, along with other tabs like "Dietary Fiber" and "Added Sugars." Do not worry about those for now. All you need to worry about is the "Total Carbohydrate" number when counting carbs.

Calories, on the other hand, are separate from carbohydrates on a nutritional facts label, though the two terms are related. A calorie is the amount of energy contained within a food. This may sound a little weird at first, but let me give you an example. Let's say a nutritional facts label on the side of an Oreo cookies box reads, "Calories: 160" and the serving size is "3 cookies"—this means that if you eat three Oreo cookies, your body will turn those cookies into 160 calories of energy. A calorie is a unit of energy. The energy (calories) from food comes from protein, fat, and carbohydrates. While fats, proteins, and carbohydrates in food all provide energy, it is predominantly carbohydrates in foods that will tend to raise the blood sugar levels in people with diabetes and therefore have to be accounted for. Some people keep a close watch on calories when they want to lose weight, but for the purposes of this book, all we need to focus on is carbs.

DO ALL CARBS ACT THE SAME WAY?

Doctors and nutritionists split carbs into two different categories: **simple carbs** and **complex carbs**. I have also heard the terms **fast carbs** and **slow carbs**. They mean the same thing—simple carbs are fast carbs, and complex carbs are slow carbs.

Simple or fast carbs are carbs that get into your system *fast*. Your body can break them down very easily because of their *simple* structure. Simple carbs will make your blood sugar spike up soon after you eat them, and then drop down rapidly once they have all been broken down. You can usually tell if something is a simple carb because it tastes really sweet. The fastest of all simple carbs are liquids, such as juice and soda. They do not need to be broken down as much as solid food when they enter your body. As a result, they can affect your blood sugars much more quickly. Here are some examples of fast carbs:

- *Juice*: any kind (apple, orange, lemonade, any of that Hi-C or Capri Sun juice, etc.)
- *Soda*: any kind, as long as it is not *diet*
- *Fruit*: apples, strawberries, oranges, mangos, and so on
- *Candy*: anything that tastes sweet and sugary (Starbursts, Skittles, Sour Patch, Mike and Ike, Nerds, Pixy Stix, etc.)
- *Syrup*: the *king* of all simple carbs—it gets into your system incredibly fast and has a lot of carbs per serving

Complex or slow carbs are basically the exact opposite of simple carbs. They are still a type of carb, so do not put these foods on the "no carb" list. However, what these foods have that simple carbs do not is substance. What I mean by substance is that the carbs in these foods will stay with you much longer than simple carbs because it takes your body a longer time to break them down (their structures are more *complex*). The longer it takes for food to get into your system, the longer it will last. As a result, these foods do not spike your blood sugar like simple carbs do. Instead of a sharp spike, the path of these carbs is more like a gradual hill. These foods commonly contain protein, fiber, and/or fat.

You tend to see complex carbs in the three big meals, breakfast, lunch, and dinner, because they provide the kind of sustenance you should be having during one of these meals. Here are some examples:

- *Pasta/Rice/Bread*: these all are commonly found in big meals and will provide your body with a carb source for hours after they are eaten

- *Potatoes*: most vegetables do not contain many carbs at all, but since potatoes are a starch, they contain a considerable amount.
- *Milk*: especially whole milk that is rich in fat
- *Bananas*: also a great source of potassium, they can help sustain your blood sugar during sporting events
- *Granola/Protein Bars*: even though they can have many different ingredients and may even contain upwards of fifty carbs, its various sources of protein help to keep the carbs sustained.

WILL MY BODY ALWAYS RESPOND TO CARBS THE SAME WAY?

No. Always keep this in mind: your body will *change*. As your body changes over the course of your life, the way you react to carbs changes too. A prime example of this is the specific period doctors call the "honeymoon phase." This phase is usually seen in people who have just been diagnosed with T1D. When someone with T1D starts receiving regular amounts of insulin right after a diagnosis, his/her pancreas will produce a little bit of insulin, too, because it is no longer under as much stress as it was before the diagnosis. Because of this "honeymoon phase," you do not have to inject a lot of insulin as your body is producing some for you. Sadly, this honeymoon phase does not last forever. It could last two weeks or two years, and doctors do not know how long any given honeymoon phase will last. When you eventually slope off and stop producing insulin altogether, the amount of insulin you will have to inject will increase. You will find yourself eating the same number of carbs but now requiring more insulin to keep your blood sugar under control. This process will happen gradually though, so don't freak out. You and your doctor will see it coming from a mile away.

Just like the honeymoon phase, your body goes through a lot of other changes that can alter the amount of insulin you need and, likewise, how you handle carbs. Age (puberty), activity, and stress are just a few examples of factors that can modify how your body responds to insulin. As I've said before, don't worry. You and your doctor will be able to adjust accordingly when the time comes.

WHAT CAN/CAN'T I EAT?

I dislike it when someone who doesn't know anything about T1D asks, "Since you have diabetes, what can and can't you eat?" It is a common misconception: that people with T1D are forbidden from eating certain foods and drinking certain drinks. You can eat and drink just about anything you want. You just have to remember to check your blood sugar and adjust how much insulin you give yourself.

When you are first diagnosed, you are most likely going to be restricted to eating between seventy and ninety carbs per meal and fifteen to thirty carbs per snack. This happened to me when I was diagnosed. I was thirteen, and all I wanted to do was eat. You have to understand that your doctors do this so they can learn about *your* T1D. Your body is going to react to carbs and insulin differently than someone else's, so your doctors need to know exactly how you handle it. Listen and trust them. Have faith in the system, and eventually, when you and your doctors understand more about your body, you will end up progressing to a more sophisticated system that allows you to be flexible with how many carbs you can eat. I know it is hard, but when you are starting out, do not eat thirty carbs over what your doctor tells you to, even if you are hungry. There are ways to soothe hunger without eating too many carbs (we will talk about ways to fill up later in this chapter).

Even though you can technically eat and drink anything you want, I will warn you that there are a few foods and drinks that, from my experience, are hard to control, even with really close management. Having a little bit of these once in a while is not going to kill you, but try not to make it a regular habit. These foods and drinks are not healthy for you anyway, so saving them for a treat is probably the best course of action. Here are the foods and drinks I have "blacklisted":

Syrup: This stuff has a crazy amount of sugar. It gets into your system really quickly and is hard to counter with insulin. The worst (and, sadly, best-tasting) syrup is the local maple syrup you find in places like Vermont. Though so delicious to put on your pancakes, it can cause blood sugar troubles. Use it sparingly or try to find a "light" version with fewer carbs.

Regular Soda: The sugar in soda also gets into your body very quickly, mainly because it is a liquid. I also find it hard to keep track of how many drinks I have when at a restaurant or anywhere with unlimited refills. Fortunately, people with T1D can choose its alternative, diet soda—it tastes just as good and has absolutely zero carbs.

Sugary Candy: If you have a sweet tooth like me, candy is a real pain to handle. On several occasions, I bought huge bags of Skittles and did not count carbs correctly when eating them. It is hard to keep track of how many handfuls of Skittles or Swedish Fish you've eaten, especially when you are just snacking while hanging with your friends. If you can successfully count carbs while snacking, more power to you; just make sure you are counting correctly. Note that even though candy is a solid food, it still falls under the "simple carb" category and will waste no time getting into your system.

Smoothies: Some of the best drinks I have ever had are smoothies. If you can find one that uses fresh fruits with no added sugar, the situation becomes much more manageable; however, some smoothies made at more popular eateries will contain added sugar. Be careful: the carbs will pile on quickly.

WHAT CAN I EAT/DRINK THAT DOES NOT HAVE MANY CARBS?

Here is a list of a few items that have between zero and ten carbs. You can have these as snacks if you cannot afford to have any more carbs, or if you are hungry but your blood sugar is high.

Food:
- *Vegetables*: Most greens and carrots have few to no carbs. Salad dressing has some carbs, but most have fewer than ten carbs

per serving. Tomatoes (technically a kind of fruit) are pretty low in carbs too.

- *Meat*: Meat is a food that fills you up *and* has no carbs. On top of that, if you eat meat along with carbs, the protein and fat in the meat will make the carbs you eat last a lot longer because the protein in the meat will slow your body's carb breakdown process.
- *Fish*: Most fish have few to no carbs, with effects similar to foods in the meat category due to high amounts of protein.
- *Eggs*: Just like meat and fish, eggs are rich in protein to help slow the body's carb breakdown process. Great for a low-carb breakfast.
- *Cheese*: Some dairy products have a substantial number of carbs, but cheese is not one of them. Cheese is a great snack food you can munch on in between meals. Be careful though—even though cheese has a small amount of carbs, it is high in calories, which is not good if you are trying to lose weight. Cheese should also be avoided if you are at risk for high cholesterol.
- *Nuts*: These are great protein-filled snacks that have very few carbs. Just make sure you are aware if you are eating some kind of trail mix that also contains M&Ms or other sweet add-ins.
- *Peanut Butter*: When you have ten scoops of peanut butter, the carbs can add up. Stick to one really big scoop or a couple of smaller ones to fill you up while still staying under the ten-carb mark (I usually count one big spoonful as about seven carbs). There are many different brands of peanut butter though, so just to be on the safe side, make sure the peanut butter you are eating does not have a lot of added sugars.
- *Gum*: Some gum can taste sweet, but one piece of gum, regardless of its taste, is never more than two carbs. It is a great alternative for people with a sweet tooth, like myself.

Drinks:

- *Water*: I've listed this just in case you did not already know: water has zero carbs.
- *Club Soda/Carbonated Water*: They both have zero carbs, which is nice in case you want to drink something that has a little more zing than just water.
- *Diet Soda*: Some people will say, "Oh no, diet soda has chemicals in it that will give you cancer; regular soda is actually better for you." Well, if you have T1D and you need to cut down on carbs, regular soda is definitely not the better choice. In the first place, any kind of soda is already not healthy for you, but all diet sodas have zero carbs. Plus, most of the time I cannot taste the difference between regular sodas and diet sodas.
- *Coffee*: If you love coffee, unless you are putting five packets of sugar and a whole lot of milk into your mug, you do not have to worry about carbs and coffee. A couple of sugar packets and a little cream will not send you over the edge, either. As a rough estimate, each sugar packet contains around 4g of carbs.
- *Tea*: On top of having basically no carbs, tea is an overall healthy drink, especially herbal and green teas. Just be mindful of the especially sweet-tasting teas. I know from personal experience that some of those "all-natural teas" with dried fruits actually contain a surprising number of carbs, so do check nutrition labels.

FIBER, FIBER, FIBER

Fiber is your friend! It can have a very real effect on how you count carbs. Eating fiber can actually allow you to eat more carbs, so keep that in mind, especially if you are on a strict carb diet. When looking at nutritional facts labels, if there is a lot of "Dietary Fiber" in the food you are eating (more than five grams), you can subtract half that amount of fiber from the "Total Carbohydrate" number on the label. For example, if you are going to eat a ham sandwich on rye bread, and the two bread slices contain six grams of fiber, you can subtract three grams of carbs from your total when tallying up the number of carbs in your sandwich. It may seem insignificant, but if you can find a way to insert fiber into your diet, it can really make a difference. Fiber is also great for people with T1D because it has that sustaining effect, similar to protein, that makes the carbs you eat alongside the fiber last longer. Fiber can also help reduce the amount of insulin you need over time. Here is a list of some foods with more than five grams of fiber (from highest to lowest amount of fiber):

- *Canned Pumpkin*: 25g per cup
- *Navy, pinto, kidney, black, lima beans, and split peas*: about 15g per cup
- *Artichokes*: 10g per artichoke
- *Prunes*: 8g per cup
- *Raspberries*: 8g per cup
- *Pears*: 5g per pear
- *Raisins*: 5g per cup
- *Rye and Wheat Bread*: 5g per two slices
- *Broccoli*: 5g per cup
- *Carrots*: 5g per cup
- *Nuts (almonds, pistachios, walnuts, peanuts, pecans, etc.)*: varies slightly, but about 5g for approximately fifty nuts
- *Oatmeal*: 8g per two cups

GOING OUT TO EAT

Going out to eat is great. You get to eat a wide variety of foods, and more times than not, it is all pretty delicious. However, since you are away from the comfort and security of your own home, you might not know off the top of your head how to handle all the carbs that are available to you. Foods at restaurants can be mysteries, even to an experienced carb counter. For example, two cheeseburgers at different restaurants can have totally different numbers of carbs. When you go out to eat, pay special attention to what you are consuming. If you have doubts about how many carbs are in front of you, just ask the waiter or waitress. If they cannot answer your question, I am sure they would be more than happy ask the chef. It is better to delay eating and double-check than to not check and give yourself the wrong amount of insulin. I have done this on several occasions, and it is not fun.

Another problem I have run into at restaurants is giving myself insulin way before the food comes out. Wait until the food is in front of you to give yourself insulin. I once gave myself insulin after I ordered, figuring it would only take fifteen to twenty minutes for the food to come out. Unfortunately, something went wrong in the kitchen that night, and it took them over an hour to serve us our food. My blood sugar dropped, and I had to drink three glasses of ginger ale to compensate.

A scenario that people do not always group into this category of "eating out" is a party. Whether it is a holiday party at someone's house or a birthday party at a local bowling alley, these situations can pose problems to people with T1D if not recognized and handled correctly. Make sure you stay on track when counting carbs, and try to account for all the snacking that you will probably do. If you decide you are going to estimate and inject a bulk amount of insulin at once so you do not have to inject every time you eat a handful of chips, I will just warn you to check your blood sugar levels often. On several occasions, I have tried to make estimates in this way and have wound up with wacky blood sugar levels because I did not check my blood sugar frequently enough.

Wherever you are, at home or out to eat, the best advice I can give you is to test your levels often and stay on top of your carb counting. If you are smart and careful, the likelihood of having abnormal blood sugar levels in any situation will be slim.

3

THOSE DARN LOW AND HIGH BLOOD SUGARS

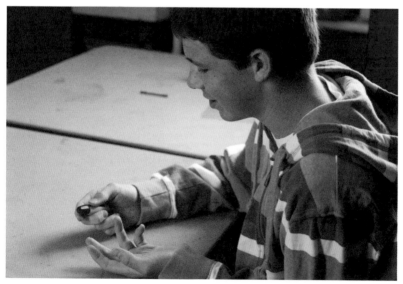

In order to learn how well you are taking care of your T1D, you need to understand your blood sugar. Your blood sugar, in plain terms, tells you how much sugar is in your blood. You do not want too much, but then again you do not want too little. This is the essence of T1D management—keep your blood sugar in the sweet spot. In order to check to see if your blood sugar is where it needs to be, you use a blood glucose meter. In this section, we will discuss what exactly your blood glucose meter tells you when it gives you a blood sugar reading, as well as what to look out for when dealing with low and high blood sugars—blood sugar levels outside the sweet spot.

DECIPHERING YOUR BLOOD GLUCOSE (BG) METER

No matter what brand or type of blood glucose (BG) meter you use, they all measure the same thing: your blood sugar. There are three main components to every BG meter kit: the machine, the test strips, and the **lancet** (finger pricker). The finger pricker is pretty self-explanatory—you use it to prick your finger to get some blood to put into the test strip. I have found that the best places to prick myself are my pinky and ring fingers, but you can get blood from any finger. Personally, I stay away from my index finger and thumb because they are more sensitive than my other fingers, and it hurts a little more when I prick them. Additionally, there are attachments to several finger prickers that allow you to get blood from your forearm. I tried this method, but I could never draw out enough blood to fill up a test strip.

The next part of the BG meter kit is the package of test strips. They usually come in bottles of fifty and are used to transfer your blood into the BG meter machine. One end of the strip is inserted into the machine while the other sticks out so you can get blood into it. Regardless of what type of test strips you use, they do not require much blood; do not squeeze your finger too tightly, thinking you need a puddle of blood for the machine to work. Once you have gotten a little bit of blood out, no more than the size of a ladybug, lightly put the tip of the test strip on the blood spot, and the strip will do the rest.

The last part of the BG meter kit is the BG meter machine. This is where the magic happens. After you let the test strip suck up some of your blood, your BG meter will beep. It takes a couple seconds, but eventually the machine will display a number on the screen. This is your blood sugar level. All BG meters in the US report blood sugar levels in the unit mg/dL (in many other countries it is reported as mmol/L). This just means that for every 1dL of your blood, there is Xmg of sugar in it. For measurement reference, there are 20dL in one two-liter bottle of soda, and a grain of salt weighs about 1mg. To put this all into perspective, if you test your blood sugar and are at the ideal blood sugar of 100mg/dL, this means that 100mg of sugar is in every 1dL of your blood. I will talk more about the meaning of these blood sugar numbers a little later in this chapter.

BG meters are becoming increasingly sophisticated with advancing technology. As a result, we are able to visualize much more than we could in the past. One of the newest features many BG meters have today is the ability to transmit your blood sugar numbers to a software program on your computer. It is fairly easy to get a cord that allows you to plug your BG meter into a computer, too, as many of them use a common micro-USB port. Once the data from your BG meter are downloaded, they can usually be organized and categorized so you can assess your blood sugar numbers over a specific duration. For example, when you look at some of the trends of your blood sugar levels, you might notice that for the past two weeks, your blood sugar has been below the sweet spot whenever you test before breakfast. Knowing this, you can talk with your doctor about changing insulin dosages to help prevent this. One of the best websites I have found for downloading and organizing my blood sugar readings is my.glooko.com. I use it all the time to make sure my blood sugar levels are on the right track.

A common question people ask is, "What BG meter is the best?" The honest answer is that no single BG meter is better than others. They all have positives and negatives, and when it really comes down to it, it's a personal choice. If someone asked me to choose a BG meter, I would say any FreeStyle BG meter. The FreeStyle test strips require a really small amount of blood to successfully get a BG reading. If you want a BG meter that is easy to carry around, OneTouch makes several BG meters that are pretty small and can easily fit into your pocket or a small bag. I used OneTouch BG meters for a long time, but when I switched to FreeStyle it was a game changer. Since FreeStyle test strips require much less blood than OneTouch test strips, I no longer have to squeeze and squeeze my fingers just to get barely enough blood to fill the test strips.

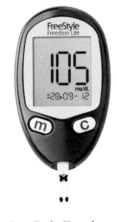

FreeStyle Freedom Lite BG meter with test strip. Printed with permission from Abbot Laboratories.

BLOOD SUGAR RANGES AND IMPORTANT NUMBERS

In this section I will discuss some key blood sugar numbers and ranges that will help you understand what those big numbers on your BG meter actually mean. In addition, I will provide some advice on how to correct your blood sugar if you are outside the sweet spot. If you have not been told this already, the normal blood sugar range a person with T1D wants to stay within is between 70 and 150—the sweet spot. Anything below 70 is considered "low," and anything above 150 is considered "high." The "low" and "high" terms mean exactly what they sound like: either you do not have enough sugar in your blood or you have too much. Besides the normal ranges we just discussed, there are certain extreme checkpoints that I also keep in my head:

- Anything **below 50** is really low. Correct your blood sugar immediately. You can technically pass out below 50, but the lowest I have ever been was 28, and I have never passed out. Do not panic if you see your BG meter give you one of these numbers, but do not waste any time correcting it, either.
- Anything **above 200**, correct with insulin. If you are below 200 (and above 150), you can usually get away with some

light exercise and drinking water to dilute the sugar in your system. If you are above 200, however, you should definitely use insulin to correct.

- Anything **above 300**, correct with insulin and check for ketones (I will explain ketones later in this chapter). Because your blood sugar levels are this high, you have to take extra caution. If you are having trouble getting rid of your high blood sugar and/or the ketones that accompany it, just call your doctor's office and they will be able to help you. Additionally, if you have a blood sugar level this high, you should probably be able to explain why: maybe you ate too much or did not take your insulin. If you are unable to explain why you are having such a high blood sugar reading, check the insulin and/or pump site you are using, as it could be faulty or not working anymore.

- There are two extremely concerning cases, both of which will be indicated on your BG meter: **"LO" and "HI."** LO means that your blood sugar is too low for the meter to read, and you should get sugar in your body immediately. Usually, LO indicates your blood sugar is **below 20**. HI is the exact opposite. This means your sugar is too high for the meter to read, at which point you should correct with insulin and definitely check for ketones. HI usually indicates your blood sugar is **above 600**. I hope you never have to see either of these messages on your BG meter screen. If you remember to count carbs and take the correct amount of insulin, there is no reason one of these should pop up on your BG meter. Having said that, if they do show up, do not panic. Just follow the appropriate correction steps and you will be fine. In these extreme cases, it might not be a bad idea to make a trip to an urgent care center or emergency room or at the very least call your diabetes doctor for help getting your blood sugar back to normal.

LOW BLOOD SUGARS VS. HIGH BLOOD SUGARS

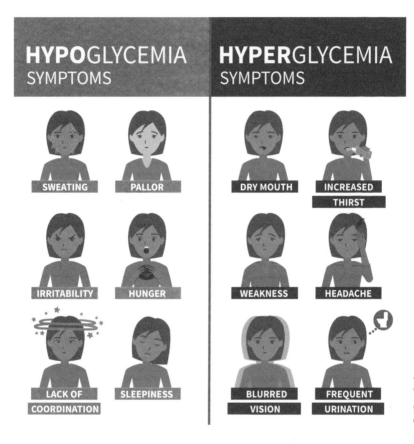

© iStockphoto

LET'S TALK ABOUT LOW BLOOD SUGARS

Low blood sugar **(hypoglycemia)** simply means you do not have
a sufficient amount of sugar in your blood. Your body needs sugar
to turn it into energy, and without enough sugar, your body cannot
sustain itself. Low blood sugars can be caused by a variety of factors, including physical activity, heat, and a surplus of insulin. Low
blood sugars affect everyone differently, and there are a multitude
of symptoms that accompany them. Here are a few: sweatiness,
light-headedness, weakness, stomachache, shakiness in the hands,
and irritability (you get angry at people for no reason). I have

experienced all of these at one point or another, and they all stink. A few days after I was first diagnosed and hospitalized, I was playing basketball in the driveway with my little sister, when all of a sudden I just felt so mad. I actually started yelling at her for no good reason. It was not until fifteen minutes after I corrected my low blood sugar that I realized what had happened. I apologized immediately, and she told me she understood. There will come a point when your blood sugar levels are so low that you can get mad at somebody for no reason, and this is unavoidable. When it happens, my advice is to apologize after you feel better. Whoever is the recipient of your short burst of rage will hopefully understand.

When you feel a low blood sugar coming on, the key steps are simple: test and rest. Sit down, drink some juice, and rest for fifteen to twenty minutes. The recommended amount of carbs for a low blood sugar correction is 16g. A glass of orange juice or a Capri Sun juice bag are my personal favorites, and each contains right around 16g of carbs. Some people also like using candy. I have used Skittles in the past, and my cousin Casey, whom I mentioned earlier in this book, carries around Starbursts (four Starbursts equal 16g of carbs, same as a juice). The only trouble with candy is that it is easy to shovel a boatload into your mouth at once, and sometimes you may eat too much only to have your blood sugar on the opposite end of the spectrum an hour later. If you are going to correct with candy, make sure you do not take more than the necessary amount. Another fan favorite is to correct low blood sugars using glucose tablets, which you can pick up in the medicine aisle of any pharmacy (my favorite flavor is sour apple). Four tablets equal 16g of carbs.

If you want my advice, I find that liquids get into my system faster than solids. Although Skittles and glucose tablets may taste really good, I know from experience that all food tastes the same when you are low. You do not really care about how food tastes; you just want the horrible feeling to go away. Liquids do not have to be broken down as much as solids and will get into your system more quickly.

In the event that you are experiencing symptoms of low blood sugar, there are rapidly-absorbed glucose (sugar) products to help avoid a diabetes emergency. They are easy-to-swallow gels that come in small packets so they can be carried with you in a pocket, purse, or bookbag. There are several brands, but I recommend the Insta-Glucose® Gel brand. I have only had to use this gel once in my life, and it worked well for me. If you are ever experiencing low blood sugar and don't respond to one of these glucose gels, I suggest strongly that you have someone bring you to the emergency room. It can be difficult to correct your blood sugar successfully when it is very low, and the people at the emergency room can really help. Better to be safe than sorry.

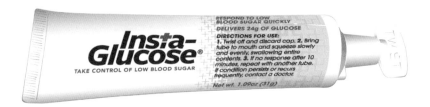

Insta-Glucose gel. © Valeant Pharmaceuticals International, Inc. Insta-Glucose is a trademark of Valeant Pharmaceuticals International, Inc. or its affiliates. The images are provided compliments of Valeant Pharmaceuticals North America, LLC; no endorsement or affiliation with the Publisher and/or Authors is implied.

Something else that is important to note, although really annoying, is that whether you drink a juice box or munch on some glucose tablets, correcting a low blood sugar is *not* an instant fix. It takes time for the sugar to get into your system, so you usually have to wait ten to fifteen minutes before you will start feeling better. After that time has passed, always recheck your blood sugar to make sure it is actually going up. On the other hand, while you are waiting out that time, do not overeat. I have caved to this urge many times in the past. All I think about is trying to get that awful "low blood sugar" feeling out of my body, and as a result I eat until the feeling goes away (i.e., nonstop eating for ten to fifteen minutes). As a result, after a couple of hours, my blood sugar is in the 300s! After you eat or drink the *correct* amount for carbs, you just have to wait it out. Take a seat, watch some TV or read a book, and be patient.

Why do I feel like this when I have low blood sugar? Isn't there a way to stop my body from feeling this way? It is important to note that the symptoms you get when you have a low blood sugar are actually really helpful. I know this sounds stupid, but think about it for a second: All of the stomach pains, headaches, dizziness, and light-headedness are your body screaming at you: "*Hey!* I need some sugar! Give me sugar!" Without these annoying notifications, how else would you know that your blood sugar is low?

Now that you understand why you get these awful symptoms, how can you prevent them from happening? Fundamentally, the more you check your blood sugar, the more you will be familiar with where your blood sugar is and where it might go. For instance, if you test your blood sugar before soccer practice and your level is seventy-five (we will talk more about sports later), you will know to drink a juice to prevent yourself from going lower as you become physically active. Exercise and physical activity are powered by the sugar in your blood. If you forget to test before practice, you will probably start feeling low twenty minutes later and will have to sit out for an extra twenty to twenty-five minutes until your blood sugar rises. I have done this many times, and I always kick myself because I know that the entire situation could have been avoided had I just tested beforehand.

Another way to avoid really low blood sugars is to treat them as soon as you feel them. If you think you feel a symptom starting but are unsure, test anyway. The sooner you know you have a low blood sugar, the sooner you can correct it. I have neglected low blood sugar symptoms before for really stupid reasons: I was doing homework, hanging with friends, or even playing soccer. For some reason, I thought that if I ignored the symptoms, they would eventually go away. I hope you understand that this is *not* how correcting a low blood sugar works. I should have listened to my body and not made up excuses to ignore it. Any excuse to not test your blood sugar is a foolish one.

> NOTE: A common place where my blood sugar has gone low is in a hot tub or jacuzzi. The heat of the water can cause your blood sugar levels to drop, so keep a sugar source next to you if you decide to take some time and relax in a hot tub or jacuzzi.

One more thing you can do to help prevent low blood sugars is review your blood sugar history either on your BG meter or on one of those websites I talked about earlier. If you notice you are always low when you wake up, talk with your doctor about reducing the amount of insulin you give yourself at night. Do not hold back from calling your doctors if you have a question or suggestion; sometimes you see things they do not. After all, you are the one who spends every second of the day with yourself and your T1D.

Emergency Glucagon Kit

Since we are on the subject of low blood sugars, let's bring up the emergency glucagon kit, encased in a bright red or orange box, which your doctors have probably given you. This kit is the last resort for low blood sugars and can end up saving your life one day. Fortunately, I have never had to use it before, and I hope I never will. If you have never had to use this instrument, I will give you the 411 on how it works. Inside every box is a daunting-looking needle filled with clear liquid. This liquid is basically water and is used as the mixing agent for the glucagon. The glucagon itself is the white powder contained within the vial next to the needle.

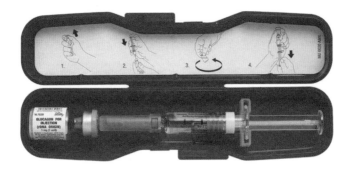

Glucagon tells your body to release sugar stored in your cells so that it can be turned into energy. The directions for using this kit are usually readily visible so that anyone can see how to use it (because odds are you will not actually be the person using this kit because you will most likely be unresponsive). You can also download the Lilly Glucagon mobile app, which will give you all the information you could possibly want or need about your glucagon kit. Just in case you want to tell someone how to use the glucagon kit so he or she can be prepared in the future, here is how it works:

1. Take the cover off the vial.
2. Take the cover off the needle, stick the needle into the vial, and push all the liquid from the needle into the vial.
3. Swirl the vial for ten to twenty seconds to mix the powder and the liquid.
4. Draw the contents from the vial back up into the needle, making sure to keep the vial upside down and the needle facing directly up (to avoid air bubbles).
5. Inject the contents into the person who needs it. Usually, the thigh is a good place to inject because it is big, tough, and hard to miss. The buttocks and the side of the stomach should also be fine.

As a person with T1D, you should own several of these glucagon kits and keep them in places you frequent. For me, I have one in my house, one in my car, and one in my backpack that I take basically everywhere with me. It is better to have too many kits than not enough. Amazingly, even though people with T1D may own multiple kits, these kits are often forgotten because most of us never have to use them. This can be dangerous because, like most things, glucagon kits have expiration dates. Make sure your kits are up to date at all times. It would be quite unfortunate if the time came when a kit needed to be used but it was not functional because it had expired. As I've mentioned, the chances of you having to use a glucagon kit is astronomically small if you take care of your T1D. Having said that, I urge you to be proactive and always stay on top of how many kits you have, where they are, and if they have expired.

LET'S TALK ABOUT HIGH BLOOD SUGARS

Put simply, **high blood sugars (hyperglycemia)** are the exact opposite of low blood sugars. When there is not enough insulin in your body, you will most likely have an excess amount of sugar in your blood. Although you might not feel the same terrible symptoms you do with low blood sugars, high blood sugars tend to produce longer-lasting effects on your body. If you have too many high blood sugars over the course of your life, your body will eventually experience problems that will not go away. An example of this is problems with your circulatory system, which can cause you to lose feeling and function in your fingers and toes. This is probably one of the scariest things that comes along with T1D. However, *do not worry*—if you take care of your T1D, you will be just fine. You will have to basically ignore the fact that you have T1D for multiple years and eat however you want for this scenario to enter the realm of possibility.

High blood sugars are most commonly caused when you eat something and forget to take insulin to cover those carbs. Sometimes you have a million things running through your head and you are not thinking about your T1D and then all of a sudden, *bam*: you are 450! This is a common mistake and has happened to me many times. It is not the end of the world, but you should correct it as soon as possible. Knowing the risks of high blood sugars, I always try especially hard to keep myself out of the high-blood-sugar range. I would rather be on the lower end of the spectrum than the higher end.

The symptoms for high blood sugars vary, but some are pretty constant across every case of T1D. Similarly, as in the case with low blood sugar symptoms, they make complete sense. Let's break it down. If you have too much sugar in your blood and not enough insulin to counteract the sugar, your body will try to do two things:

1. Flush as much of the excess sugar out of your body as possible
2. Dilute your body with water to minimize the concentration of the sugar, as well as replace the water that is being used to flush out the excess sugar.

This is why common symptoms for high blood sugars are thirst, dry mouth, and frequent urination. You urinate to flush the excess sugar out of your body, which then causes thirst because you need to replace the water you just lost. The dry mouth symptom comes into play because your body pulls water from everywhere when trying to flush out the sugar, including your saliva (which has a lot water in it). If you cannot already see the pattern, it looks like this: pee . . . drink . . . pee . . . drink . . . pee . . . drink . . . . This process is a cycle, and it does not end until you correct your blood sugar. Other symptoms that can arise if you have high blood sugar for a long time are weakness, blurry vision, and dizziness, all of which are common symptoms associated with dehydration. Hmmm . . . I wonder why that is?

The symptoms I just mentioned, with the addition of rapid weight loss, are probably symptoms similar to what you experienced before diagnosis. Before you were diagnosed, you were not taking insulin because you did not know you had T1D. Consequently, you constantly had high blood sugars. The reason for the weight loss is that your body was not getting any sugar from your blood because you had no insulin, so it started looking for energy in other places. In the absence of insulin, your body can't get glucose into its cells, so it tries to compensate by making a lot of new sugar. It does this by breaking down your stores of fats and proteins and converting these building blocks into sugar in the liver. The liver then dumps all of this sugar into the bloodstream, where it builds up even higher and gets removed from your body in the urine. The weight loss comes from the loss of these important fat and muscle stores—you are literally peeing them away. One of my friends who was diagnosed with T1D when he was just ten years old lost over twenty pounds in two weeks from this process!

Common terms associated with high blood sugar levels are **ketones** and **diabetic ketoacidosis (DKA)**. They both refer to the same thing: When your body starts breaking down fat for glucose because you have no insulin and cannot get sugar from your blood, ketones are produced in the process. Ketones enter your blood and eventually spill over into your urine. Ketones are acids, and they can cause dangerous chemical imbalances in both your blood and urine. This is why when you test for ketones, you pee on a little stick, which will tell you if your urine is acidic or not (kind of like those sticks you put into a pool to test the various chemical levels). It is always good to test for ketones if you think your blood sugar has been running high for a long time. If you do have DKA, it is not an emergency, but you should call your doctor so he or she can help you get back on track. Getting rid of ketones can be a little trickier than just taking care of a high blood sugar, but you must try your very best to remove them. The last thing you want is a bunch of free-flowing acid moving throughout your body. Another important note about DKA is that you can get them even if you

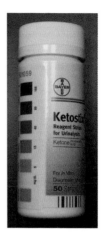

Bayer Ketostix bottle. Used
with permission from Ascensia
Diabetes Care (Bayer).

do not have high blood sugars. If you have absolutely no insulin
in your body, even if you only have a blood sugar of, say, 150, you
may start to develop ketones. This is a common occurrence when
people with T1D get sick since they do not eat much during a
sickness, which causes them to take significantly less insulin, if
any at all (we will talk about how to handle T1D and sickness as
well as how DKA can sometimes mask itself as sickness in chapter
5, "Stupid Sick Days").

So how do you correct a high blood sugar? Well, first, drink
water. When you have high a blood sugar, your body wants water
for a reason. Help the process along. Physical activity can also
help lower your blood sugar. You use up more sugar when you are
physically active, so reduce your high blood sugar level by turning
some of it into energy. Running, swimming, biking, and about a
million other activities will do the trick. Just be careful that you
are not participating in a physical activity that will be negatively
impacted by your high blood sugar. Performing physical activities
confidently can vary from person to person, but regardless, know
your limits and what you can do safely while also "under the spell"
of any high blood sugar symptoms. One time I tested my blood
sugar and I was 300, so I figured I would ride my bike a little to burn
off some of the sugar. Once I got out of my driveway, I started to

feel dizzy and immediately fell off my bike once I got on the road (not a smart move!).

The best thing you can do to correct any high blood sugar is to take insulin. If your body is freaking out because you do not have any insulin, you should probably give it some. How much insulin to take can be tricky, though. The amount of insulin to give someone based on how high his or her blood sugar is varies from person to person. You and your doctor will have certain correction ratios set up so you can successfully correct your blood sugar. For example, I give myself one unit of insulin for every 30mg/dL I am above 150. So if I am 323, which is close to 330, I would give myself seven units of insulin: starting from 150, 323 is about seven sets of 30mg/dL higher than 150 (150, 180, 210, 240, 270, 300, 330).

Now, for the prevention part. This is going to sound dumb, but since the most common mistake made by people with T1D that causes high blood sugar levels is forgetting to take insulin, the best solution is to remember to take your insulin. It sounds simple, but I had trouble with this for years, and still do on occasion. I do not do it on purpose; I just forget sometimes. What has helped me immensely is to set alarms around the times I think I am going to be eating each of my main meals. Even if the alarm happens to be thirty minutes off from when I actually eat, it is still a good reminder. Another important factor to check to see what could be causing your high blood sugar is your insulin. Make sure that the insulin you are using has not expired or degraded. Extreme heat, like on a day at the beach, can cause your insulin to stop working. Similarly, if you use an insulin pump, double-check your pump and pump site (we will talk about pumps in chapter 4, "Insulin on All Fronts: Injections and Pumps"). Make sure your pump is still turned on and is not in "suspend" mode. Likewise, double-check to make sure your pump site is securely on your body. If you just played in a sporting event or you toss and turn when you sleep, you can hit the site and cause it to stop putting insulin into your body.

CONTINUOUS GLUCOSE MONITOR (CGM)

The continuous glucose monitor (CGM) is a revolutionary way to keep track of your blood sugar levels. The CGM does exactly what it says—it continuously monitors your blood sugar. It is composed of two main parts: the sensor and the receiver. The sensor is a small semispherical machine no bigger than a small strawberry. It sticks directly to your body and needs to be changed roughly once every seven days. A small sensor is inserted right under the skin to constantly record your blood sugar (usually once every five minutes). Those blood sugar readings are then relayed wirelessly to the receiver, which you can keep anywhere on your person, such as in a backpack or a pocket. With some CGMs, you can also download an app on your phone and computer that displays the data collected from the receiver. I have personally never used a CGM, but many of my friends have, and I am seriously considering it in the near future.

There are several advantages to using a CGM. The first is that while you still need to test your blood sugar the regular way a couple of times every day to calibrate the CGM and make sure it is reading accurate blood sugar levels, you will not need to prick your fingers as often as you typically would. On top of that, since the CGM is constantly taking your blood sugar, it is very easy to see trends. When you test your blood sugar normally, all you get is a number with absolutely no indication of whether your blood sugar is going up or down. With the CGM, however, you know which direction your blood sugar is trending and at what rate. This is really helpful if you are trying to decide how to correct a blood sugar outside of the sweet spot. For example, if your blood sugar is 215, you might be on the fence about correcting with insulin or just some water and physical activity. But when you look at your CGM and it shows that your last two blood sugar readings were 250 and then 225, you can easily see that your blood sugar is currently trending downward, and taking insulin is thus not necessary.

Additionally, you can set specific alarms on your CGM to warn you if your blood sugar is too high or low or is trending too quickly in either direction. From what I have heard, the only annoying part about using a CGM are these alarms, which can start to pester you really quickly. Personally, I think a couple of alarms are a small price to pay for excellent blood sugar control.

I have heard of two brands of CGMs in my discussions with friends who have T1D. The first is Dexcom. This is the more popular one in my experience, and it keeps improving. It is very slim and sleek, and a lot of my more active friends with T1D use and love it. Another great feature about the Dexcom CGMs is the fact that they can sync to iPhones, so your blood sugar and trends are never more than a swipe away. One of my friends with T1D even has her Dexcom CGM, the G5 model, linked to an app she downloaded on her Apple watch. How amazing is that? Dexcom CGMs can also link with certain insulin pumps, like the t:slim X2.

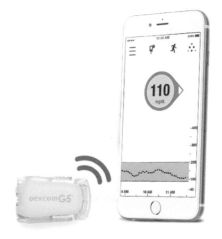

Dexcom G5 with associated phone application. Used with permission from Dexcom, Inc.

The other brand I am familiar with is Medtronic. Medtronic has a lot more products than Dexcom and can therefore offer a wider range of customization. Additionally, Medtronic makes insulin pumps, so their CGMs can sync with insulin pumps to create a **hybrid closed-loop system** or **artificial pancreas** (I will discuss insulin pumps and how they work with CGMs in chapter 4, "Insulin on All Fronts: Injections and Pumps").

The CGM is an initial time commitment because it requires a lot of careful attention and focus when starting out. You have to calibrate it and listen for when its alarms go off, but if you really want to keep control of your blood sugar levels, this is the way to go.

THE MAIN SCOOP

There is a lot of information in this chapter about many different topics. The best tip I can give to you for avoiding both low and high blood sugars is to stay aware of your T1D. It can be a pain sometimes, but it sure beats the heck out of feeling terrible and then having to spend a bunch of time trying to correct a mistake that could have been easily avoided. Stay on top of it the best you can. There will come times when you will have to correct both high and low blood sugars, so just recall the right methods to use, and do not get angry with yourself. No one is perfect . . . even us people with T1D.

4

INSULIN ON ALL FRONTS: INJECTIONS AND PUMPS

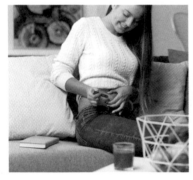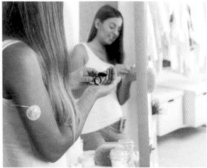

Insulin is without a doubt the most important part of T1D management. We have to supply our bodies with insulin because our pancreas no longer produces it. But *how* and *what kind* of insulin you put into your body varies greatly. I have experienced both daily injections, consisting of many different types of insulin, as well as insulin pumps, and I will discuss and compare them in this chapter.

The first important item to note is how to keep any insulin in your possession from going bad (degrading). Insulin is a pretty stable medication, but if it is left in an area that is too cold or too hot, it can lose its potency and will not work when you want it to.

When you get insulin, it is best to keep it chilled. Insulin should be kept in a refrigerator (not freezer) before it is opened, and once opened it can stay at room temperature (but I still keep mine in the fridge). You can keep it in your pocket or in a backpack, but do not leave your backpack in a 100°F car all day or under a towel at the beach. Another good tip that helps me keep track of my insulin is to keep it all in one place. Back when I was diagnosed, I used three different types of insulin, and sometimes it was hard to keep track of it all. Designate a spot in your refrigerator for "insulin only." This might also be an opportunity to ask your parents if you can have a minifridge for your bedroom. You didn't hear it from me, but this is one of those instances where T1D might help you out . . . take advantage of it.

DAILY INJECTIONS

Almost everyone who is diagnosed with T1D starts insulin treatments by **daily injections**. When your doctor is trying to figure out how your body responds to insulin and carbs, this method is the best because it can be easily modified and tweaked to fit your body. People on daily injections also have the benefit of not having an insulin pump attached to them 24/7. However, there are drawbacks too. Since you do not have your insulin attached to you as you would with a pump, you have to carry it around wherever you go. If you do not like needles, this method can also prove difficult because you will have to take multiple injections every day. Additionally, you have to keep track of all your different types of insulin. In this next section, I will go over each type of insulin, what it does, and a couple of basic regimens of daily injections. The colors in parentheses indicate the color casing each type of insulin is wrapped in. The insulins will be listed from fastest acting to slowest acting.

Types of Insulin

NovoLog/Humalog (orange/maroon): This is your fast-acting insulin. You take this to cover any food you are eating at that moment. For instance, if you are about to have a sandwich, you would take a certain amount of NovoLog or Humalog to cover however many carbs are in the pizza. This is also the type of insulin that is used to fill insulin pumps. When on a pump, this is normally the only type of insulin you are taking. Do not get confused by the names either—NovoLog and Humalog act the same way and are only slightly different molecules.

Humulin N/Novoin N (NPH) (yellow/lime green/orange): This type of insulin is usually taken in the morning in order to cover carbs that will be eaten later in the day. It takes a while to kick in and then peaks hours after it is taken. People commonly take this at breakfast with the intention of covering the carbs they will have at lunch. A cool thing about this insulin is that it can be mixed with NovoLog, so you can combine the two into one syringe at breakfast and save yourself from taking two injections in the morning. The drawback is that if you take this insulin, you are committing yourself to eating a specific number of carbs at lunchtime. If you take twenty units of NPH to cover eighty carbs at lunch, you have to make sure you eat eighty carbs at lunch—no more, no less. You and your doctors will decide which NPH is right for you, should you decide to use it.

Levemir (green): In people who do not have T1D, the pancreas always produces some insulin to keep the liver from

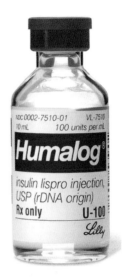

Eli Lilly Humalog vial. © Eli Lilly and Company. All rights reserved. Used with permission.

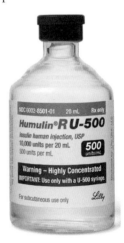

Eli Lilly Humulin R U-500 vial. © Eli Lilly and Company. All rights reserved. Used with permission.

overproducing glucose. This is known as basal insulin. Levemir is a long-acting basal insulin that is usually taken once a day in the evening or twice a day before breakfast and dinner. It is used to regulate your blood sugar levels between meals and during the overnight period when you are sleeping.

Lantus (light purple): This is another basal insulin that may last even longer than Levemir. This is usually taken once a day at bedtime and will sustain blood sugar over twenty-four hours. This insulin is a nice alternative to Levemir because you can take one Lantus injection per day instead of two Levemir injections. However, if you take two injections of Levemir, you may have more control as you can change how much insulin to give yourself at the halfway point of your twenty-four-hour period. With Lantus, on the other hand, you can only make insulin adjustments at one time during your twenty-four-hour period since you are taking only one injection per day. Keep in mind that you are not supposed to mix either of these long-acting insulin with NovoLog or Humalog.

Lantus insulin pen. Used with permission from Sanofi.

Different Regimens

There are different combinations of insulins you can use to manage your T1D. The plan I started out with entailed an injection of NovoLog and NPH in the morning, followed by two injections at dinner, one of NovoLog and one of Levemir. This plan calls for a set number of carbs per meal (usually somewhere between forty and ninety carbs based on age, size, and gender). It is a great plan to start on because it keeps your daily intake of both insulin and carbs constant. As a result, it is easy to find out how your body responds to insulin and carbs. This is why my doctors use this regimen as a starting point for their patients with T1D.

Once my doctors and I understood how my body reacted to insulin and carbs, I switched insulin regimens to a plan that entailed two injections of Levemir per day, one at breakfast and one at dinner, and then individual injections of NovoLog whenever I ate. This plan allowed me to eat whatever and whenever I wanted as long as I accounted for the carbs and took the right amount of NovoLog. The drawback of this plan was that I had to inject myself whenever I wanted to eat, which became kind of annoying. As I mentioned before, a modification to this regimen could be to drop the two Levemir injections and simply take one Lantus injection to sustain you for over twenty-four hours. I do not mind taking injections, so I decided on the regimen that would give me the most control.

How and Where to Inject

Injections can sometimes be a pain, but if you know how and where to inject, they can actually be quite easy, and more important, painless. The first tip about injecting yourself is to not repeatedly inject yourself in the same spot. This will cause the tissue where you inject to become hard—eventually so hard that insulin will not be absorbed into the blood stream as well. This has happened to me—and it stinks. Because the insulin cannot get through your tissue, a hard bubble of insulin forms between the layers of tissue. Once developed, it takes a while for this hard tissue to go away—sometimes months. The lesson to be learned here is to always rotate where you inject yourself. When I was on daily injections, I formed a pattern to make sure I was always injecting myself in different places (left stomach, right stomach, left arm, right arm). If you forget where you injected yourself last, just feel your skin and make sure you are not injecting into a spot that feels kind of hard.

Another important tip that commonly gets overlooked is wiping the spot you are going to inject with an alcohol wipe. Besides the fact that using an alcohol wipe will help prevent bacterial infections,

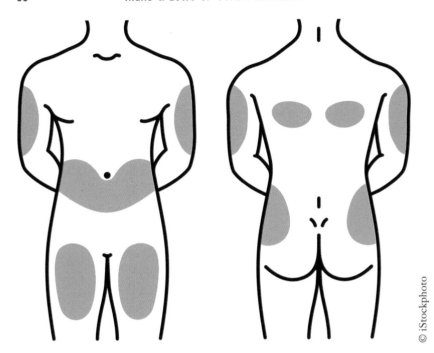

I also find that it helps my skin heal from those little repeated injections. Alcohol wipes can be bought in any pharmacy and are very cheap, so do not sell yourself short by not using them. I am sure your parents would be more than happy to purchase some if you ask.

Let's talk about *where* to inject yourself. The goal of the game here is less pain. No one, including people with T1D, wants to experience pain. To avoid as much pain as possible, we have to find places on our bodies where the pain of injecting is minimal, and the best places to inject are the fattiest ones. Everyone has at least a little fat on their bodies (except perhaps marathon runners or Olympic athletes, in which case I salute you), so you just have to find those spots for injections. The best places for me are the stomach (front and side), the side of the arm, and the upper thighs. Some people also inject in the side part of their buttocks. A good tip I learned to make sure I am injecting into fat is to prop up or pinch the fat at the location of injection. For my arms, I prop the fat up using the corner of a doorway. Turn your arm so it is facing the corner of the doorway, place your arm lightly on the corner, and then slightly drag your arm down the corner to prop up any fat that is present. When I inject in my stomach I use the pinching method. Pinch the skin so there is about an inch of space in between your fingers, and then inject into that space. It helps to be seated when you do this too because it compresses all the skin and fat in your stomach area. This method works extremely well and, on occasion, can be absolutely pain-free.

Here's another tip about injecting big doses of insulin—like thirty units of Levemir at suppertime. When you inject a big dose of insulin all at once, it hurts sometimes. I think it is probably because you are sending so much insulin through your tissue at once. The pain associated with it feels like an intense burning sensation under the skin. If you want to avoid this sensation, inject half of the dose and wait a couple of seconds before injecting the rest. Alternatively, you can also try injecting the whole insulin dose extra slowly to minimize the pain.

Daily Injections Summary

As I have mentioned, an advantage to using the daily injection method is not having anything attached to you at all times, like a pump. However, the tradeoff is you have to take multiple injections every day. I was on daily injections for almost eight years following my diagnosis, including almost two years of college, and I never felt overwhelmed. One of my father's friends, Jimmy, has successfully managed daily injections for decades, while also working as an elite Division I football referee. Not too shabby! My point in telling you this is that it is possible to stay on daily injections for your entire life. Some people prefer daily injections and can lead very healthy lives while on it. However, as you progress through your years of T1D, you may find many people, including your doctors, pushing you to try an insulin pump. One of my Yale doctors conducted the first study that showed that insulin pumps really worked; as a result they were always pushing pump therapy. It is generally known as a more sophisticated way of managing your T1D, and people on pumps generally have better control over their blood sugar levels. This is *not* a sales pitch, and I am *not* trying to force you to use a pump. However, I would advise you to at least try it out at some point in your life. No harm can come from testing a different insulin management method. And who knows, maybe you will like it better than you initially thought.

INSULIN PUMP

Using an **insulin pump** has some fundamental similarities and differences to daily injections. Let's go through the similarities, and then we will talk about the differences that often sway people to switch to the insulin pump.

- **Same type of insulin:** Just because you are switching systems does not mean you are putting something completely different into your body. Most pump patients fill their insulin pumps with NovoLog or Humalog, since they work so much alike.

- **You still count carbs:** Having an insulin pump does not allow you to forget about counting carbs. On the contrary, having a pump is completely dependent on putting the right amount of insulin into your body based on both your blood sugar level and how many carbs you are taking in.

- **You still have to test your blood:** The only thing an insulin pump does is give you insulin. Some of the pumps act as BG meters as well, and some are also able to sync with a continuous glucose monitor (CGM) (we will discuss specific insulin pumps later in this section). For the most part, however, you still have to manually input your blood sugar levels into your pump after testing your blood sugar with your regular BG meter.

Although similar in several key ways, an insulin pump is a whole new way to manage your T1D. Although you always have something attached to you, which some people do not like because it feels like a T1D "label," the pump allows you to be much more flexible with how you live your life. I am a big advocate of the insulin pump, and everyone should try it. I find it is a *lot* easier to control my blood sugar levels with an insulin pump. Let's go over the basic mechanisms of a typical insulin pump, before we go into more detail with some specifics about the different pumps on the market.

Infusion Site and Pump

An insulin pump is composed of a couple of main parts: the **pump** and the **infusion catheter**, which connects to the body at the infusion site. The pump contains a mini-computer, which regulates the infusion of insulin, which is stored in a reservoir in the pump. The outlet of the insulin reservoir in the pump is connected to a tube called the **cannula**. The other end of the cannula is connected to the infusion site that includes a needle through the skin, which is the path the insulin takes to get into your body. The pump and cannula can be disconnected (and easily reconnected) from the infusion site, just in case you need to disconnect the pump for things like swimming or sports. In some newer insulin pumps, the insulin is kept in a pod that is attached directly to the site without the need for the cannula. In this type of pump, the insulin infusion from the pod is regulated by a handheld device. Just like an insulin injection, you want to put the site in a fatty place so it does not hurt when it goes in or when you move around. Normally, you have to replace the site once every two to three days, which is a huge improvement from multiple injections every single day.

As I mentioned in the section on daily injections, use alcohol wipes on the place where you are going to put your site to prevent bacterial infections. Using alcohol wipes to sterilize your pump site area is much more important than it is for daily injections because your pump site is always in your body, and the area needs to be sterilized as it is constantly open and exposed. I had never used alcohol wipes until one summer when I put a pump site on—when I took it off after three days, the site was red and sensitive to the touch. I left it alone for a week, but the area kept getting bigger and bigger, and I actually started feeling sick. I eventually had to go to an urgent care unit to get examined. The doctor told me I had gotten a skin infection and prescribed antibiotics for me to take for a few weeks. Ever since then, I make sure a pump site never touches a part of my body that has not been cleaned with an alcohol wipe.

Where can I put my insulin site? A pump site is very similar to a daily injection in the sense that you want to find a fatty spot to use as your site of injection, like your stomach, arm, thigh, or side of your buttocks. If your site is attached to your pump by a tube, putting the site on your arm is out of the question. The tube (cannula) that connects the infusion site to the pump comes in several different lengths (18, 23, 32, and 43 inches), but nevertheless it can be highly restricting and annoying if attached to your arm (since you usually keep the pump in your pants pocket). Oh, and just to answer this question you probably have: *no*, you cannot feel the infusion site catheter that pierces the skin when it is inside of you. You can ask anyone you know who has a pump, and they will all say that most of the time they forget they even have it on. One last tip: Be careful if you decide to put your infusion site on your thigh. Placing it below the belt line can sometimes be dangerous because you can rip the site when you pull your pants down, and I have done this many times. It kind of hurts when it gets ripped off, but it annoys me more than anything else because I realize the only reason it has happened is because I forgot about it. Additionally, I sometimes find it hard to avoid muscle when putting an insulin site on my thigh. You will most likely know if you hit muscle when the cannula goes into your leg (as it will definitely hurt), and you will have to rip the site out and try somewhere else with a new site. The thigh can be an excellent place to put your insulin site because your clothing will always cover it up; just be mindful of the drawbacks that come with it.

The second part of the insulin pump is the mini-computer that regulates insulin delivery. It is the part of the pump you give commands to. You tell it what your blood sugar is, how many carbs you are going to eat, and sometimes how much insulin to inject. Most pumps run on AAA-batteries, so always make sure you have a few on-hand in case your pump suddenly shuts down. The great thing about the modern pumps is that most, if not all, of them have settings you can input that will help you calculate the right amount of insulin to give for any situation. Let's talk a little about each of these settings.

I:C Ratio and Correction Factor Ratio

When going on an insulin pump, you and your doctor will come up with ratios that are specific to your body. Most likely you will already have an idea of what these ratios are based on calculations you performed when giving daily injections (you probably just didn't know their formal names). These ratios include your **insulin-to-carb (I:C) ratio** and your **correction factor ratio**. Your I:C ratio is simply the amount of carbs you can eat for every 1 unit of insulin. For preteens it can be as much as 20 grams of carb for every 1 unit of insulin; whereas in adolescents the insulin-to-carb ratio is usually 1 unit of insulin for every 10 grams of carbs (or even less). For example, the typical teenager with an I:C ratio of 1:10 who wants to eat 60 grams of carbs for breakfast would take 6 units of insulin (one unit for every 10 grams) before breakfast.

Just like the I:C ratio, the correction factor is different for everyone, and it changes over time. What the correction factor tells you is how much insulin you need to take to correct a high blood sugar level. As an example, let's say you need to take 1 unit of insulin for every 30mg/dL your blood sugar is above 150, and your blood sugar level is 330. In this case, you need to take 6 units of insulin to correct for the high blood sugar level. Here is how this insulin dose was calculated: the actual blood sugar level (330) minus the target blood sugar level (150) equals 180; 180 divided by the correction factor (30) equals 6 units. The correction factor is most often used when the blood sugar level is too high before the meal. If that's the case, using the I:C ratio alone probably won't get you back to target before the next meal. You need a little extra insulin to get near to target.

The I:C ratio and correction factor are very important because they make sure you are not giving yourself too much or too little insulin. One of the great things about the insulin pump is that once you plug these ratios into the pump's computer, the computer will do all the calculations for you. You do not have to know, for instance, that if you are 210 and are going to have fifty carbs, you have to give yourself 7.80 units of insulin. All you have to do is test your blood sugar and count how many carbs you are going to eat, and then plug both those numbers into your pump. It will do the rest. Pretty sweet, right? The other great part is that the pump can accurately deliver small fractions of a unit of insulin, which is not possible with daily insulin injections.

The last important setting you need to know about is your basal rate. When on daily injections, you either took one injection of Lantus or two injections of Levemir every day. These insulins help stabilize your blood sugar levels. You still need that stability with an insulin pump, but now you do not have either of those insulins at your disposal. As a better alternative, insulin pumps can be programmed to infuse small amounts of fast-acting insulin throughout your day, and what is more, this amount can be changed every thirty minutes. The preprogrammed amount that you receive from the pump is called your basal rate. Unlike the last two settings that were similar to calculations you performed when on daily injections, the basal rate setting is a completely new calculation, so it might take you and your doctor a little longer to find the basal amount of insulin that is right for you.

Most insulin pumps should also have a port that you can plug into your computer to retrieve all the data stored in the pump's computer. These data include your blood sugar levels, carbs inputted, and insulin delivered. There are software programs that work with certain pumps too. When you plug your pump into your computer, the software will take the data, organize them, and even spit out cool graphs. You and your doctor can use this to track your blood sugars and see trends that you otherwise might not have seen. My favorite software program to use for organizing and visualizing my data, which I have mentioned earlier in this book, is my.glooko.com.

Specific Insulin Pumps

Before I start this section, I want to make you aware that insulin pump brands are constantly updating and upgrading their products. To find the most up-to-date hardware and software for insulin pumps, check various insulin pump brand websites and even with your diabetes doctor.

There are many different types of insulin pumps that have different abilities and features on top of the more general functions I have just discussed. Here are a few different pump brands and models with some unique features:

Insulet OmniPod: This is the pump I am currently using, and *I love it*. The pump itself is tubeless, so there is no foot-long cannula to worry about. Because of this, I have the freedom to put the site in more places than usual, like my arms. Just as a tip: Whenever I put the site on my arm, I usually wear one of those athletic compression sleeves, commonly made out of spandex material, in order to hold it in place. The separate handheld device that regulates the OmniPod pump (called the PDM) also includes a BG meter, which communicates directly with the mini-computer in the PDM. Instead of inputting your blood sugar levels manually, you can put FreeStyle test strips into a port in the PDM to test your blood sugar. After you test, the number automatically goes into the PDM's computer and can be readily used for insulin calculations.

Medtronic: This pump brand is great because they offer many options, including the MiniMed 530G, MiniMed 630G, and

MiniMed 670G insulin pumps (530G being the oldest and 670G being the newest). The MiniMed 670G system is also compatible with the Guardian Sensor 3 (a CGM) to help and even correct your blood sugar levels (I discussed CGMs in chapter 3: "Those Darn Low and High Blood Sugars"). This system is called a **hybrid closed-loop system**, also known as an **artificial pancreas**. Essentially, the CGM reads your blood sugar every five minutes and relays those numbers to your pump, which then changes your basal rate of insulin based the blood sugar readings from the CGM. If your blood sugar is too low, the pump will temporarily lower or shut off your basal dose of insulin until your blood sugar has recovered. Similarly, if your blood sugar is high, the pump will temporarily increase your basal dose of insulin. You still have to calibrate the CGM and manually input carbohydrates when you want to eat, but the fact that these two machines can work together is unbelievable. In my eyes, this is the future of T1D: a system that actively seeks to help you keep your blood sugar levels within a comfortable range.

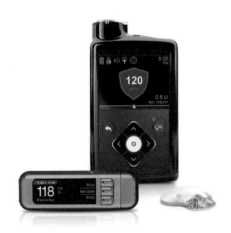

Medtronic 670 G insulin pump with Guardian Sensor 3 CGM. Used with permission from Medtronic.

Tandem: There are currently three different models of Tandem brand pumps (t:slim X2, t:slim G4, and t:flex). The software on these pumps is really colorful and user friendly. The pumps are also touchscreens, which some people prefer over regular buttons. Most pumps use batteries, but these pumps charge as well, so you will never have to worry about it suddenly and unexpectedly dying (as long as you charge it regularly). Each model is pretty similar to the others with just a few minor differences. The t:flex has the capacity to hold more insulin, while the t:slims are known for being quite thin and easy to travel with. The t:slim X2 is the newest and most modern model, but the t:slim G4 has the ability to link with a Dexcom CGM in order to clearly show you blood sugar levels alongside insulin doses. Note: Do not get this confused with the hybrid closed-loop system seen with Medtronic pumps. With Tandem pumps, the information is only displayed together; the numbers recorded from the Dexcom CGM *do not* influence the insulin given by the t:slim G4.

Animas: Although I have never used this brand of pump, nor have any of my friends, I have received very positive feedback from diabetes doctors and medical professionals. This pump brand has two models, the Vibe and the OneTouch Ping. The Vibe displays data extremely well, which makes looking at blood sugar trends easy, and it is compatible with the Dexcom G4. The OneTouch Ping syncs wirelessly with a BG meter, so when you test your blood sugar, the readings will be automatically relayed to the pump.

SO . . . DAILY INJECTIONS OR INSULIN PUMP?

The choice to use daily injections or an insulin pump is completely up to you. Some people do better with one, while others do better with the other. Know your body and what you think would help you control your T1D best. If you have been on the same plan for a long time and your blood sugar levels are starting to go wacky, try another system. You can always return to the one you used before if something does not work. Talk with your diabetes doctors about your options and ask them what they think is the best option for you. Having said that, do not let anyone, including your doctors, force you into a system you are uncomfortable with. You know your body and what it needs better than anyone else on the planet.

5

STUPID SICK DAYS

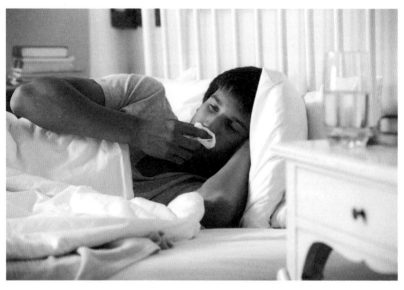

Getting sick stinks, regardless of whether you have T1D or not. You feel terrible, and you really cannot do anything except rest and wait to get better. Unfortunately, having T1D means you have to pay attention to a few other things on top of actually being sick. In this chapter, I will describe how exactly to take care of your T1D when feeling under the weather. Note: If this topic is still kind of new to you and some of the things discussed in this chapter still do not make sense, the best thing to do is to call your doctor's office. Your doctor will be able to help you through your sickness with ease. A lot of diabetes doctors actually prefer that you call them when you are sick just so they can make sure everything goes smoothly.

When you know you are sick, one of the best things you can do to control your T1D is to test your blood sugar frequently. Test, test, test! It can be annoying (believe me, I know), but you have to do it in order to keep your blood sugar where it needs to be. Setting alarms to remind yourself to test is crucial when you are sick. On several occasions when I was sick, I took NyQuil to sleep and woke up eight hours later to find my blood sugar in the 300s. Alarms are perfect because they wake you up just long enough so you can test your blood sugar and adjust if needed.

Another thing you have to do is to check for DKA (we talked about ketones in chapter 3, "Those Darn Low and High Blood Sugars"). When you are sick, you usually refrain from eating a lot and, thus, take less insulin. Since DKA arises when you do not have enough insulin in your body, you are much more susceptible to ketones when you are sick. Remember: DKA can arise even if your blood sugar is normal. Testing for DKA is another pain-in-the-butt thing you have to do that is essential for successful T1D management, especially when you are sick.

Sometimes it can be hard to eat when you are sick. You do not feel well, your stomach aches, and you already feel nauseous . . . who wants to eat when they feel like that? If you do not plan on eating a lot, it is okay to back off on how much insulin you give yourself, but you should definitely check with your diabetes doctor before doing this.

Sometimes, you will eat food when you are sick but your body may not want to keep it down. Consequently, you vomit it back up. If you are vomiting and you are not sure what your blood sugar is doing, test immediately. I would also advise calling your doctors and letting them know. If you test your blood sugar and find that you are low, say 56, this would be the time to use that Insta-Glucose gel I talked about in chapter 3, "Those Darn Low and High Blood Sugars." Rub this gel on the inside of your gums and the sugar will absorb into the skin of your gums—no swallowing necessary. Keep an extra-close eye on your blood sugar levels and make sure they return to normal. This happened to me once, and on top of using the Insta-Glucose gel, I decided it was a good idea to go to the emergency room. I understood that I could not control my own blood sugar, so I told my mom, and she drove me to the ER to get things back under control.

This last piece of advice is sometimes hard to apply, especially for someone who is independent, like myself: It is okay to ask for help from a friend or parent. Tell them that you are sick and that you need their help to make sure your blood sugar levels stay on track. Ask people you know and trust. Allow them to wake you up, test your blood sugar, and give you insulin. It can be difficult to remember everything you have to do when you are sick, T1D related or not, so having at least one other person helping you is never a bad idea.

DIABETIC KETOACIDOSIS
Wearing the Mask of SicknessDiabetic ketoacidosis (DKA), which I explained earlier in chapter 3, "Those Darn Low and High Blood Sugars," is a condition where your body overproduces ketones, which makes your blood acidic (lower pH). It is also accompanied by symptoms such as stomachaches, nausea, and vomiting—symptoms someone might associate with being sick. People with T1D are susceptible to DKA because they don't make enough insulin to keep their bodies from overproducing ketones, and they are especially susceptible at times of physical or emotional stress because the amount of insulin they are taking may not be enough to suppress ketone production. People who are on insulin pumps are particularly vulnerable to developing DKA, since they often will not receive any warning that they are not getting any insulin if their infusion set has clogged or kinked. The first red-flag that people who use

insulin pumps may receive is that blood sugar levels remain high despite taking a correction dose of insulin. If this happens, you have to put in a new infusion set and may need to take a correction dose by injection rather than by the pump. Regardless of the method that you use to take insulin, always remember that if your stomach aches, if you feel nauseous, or if you have thrown up, you have to check for ketones.

MENSTRUATION

For all you women out there, I want to discuss briefly how your menstrual cycle can affect your T1D. I know you are not technically sick when you are menstruating, but your T1D management can be affected because of this temporary physical change, which is why I decided to include it in this chapter.

My personal experience on this matter is nonexistent, but I have discussed this topic with several of my female friends who have T1D. The most common factor I have discovered between menstruation and T1D is that there is no common factor. Some women I have talked with have said that they see absolutely no changes in their blood sugar levels when they are on their periods, while others say it affects them greatly.

Several women have told me that they notice their blood sugar levels rise a couple of days prior to their period. I have done some research on this and, as it turns out, your body produces a lot of hormones, namely estrogen and progesterone, a few days before your period. These hormones can affect your blood sugar levels by affecting the insulin you put into your body. According to published reports, your blood sugar levels will return to normal when your period begins, so you mainly have to stay alert for those couple of days before.

Just like anything else involving T1D, effects can vary greatly from person to person. Talk with your doctors, and they will help you find the best way to manage your T1D alongside your menstrual cycle.

6

GOING TO YOUR DOCTOR'S OFFICE

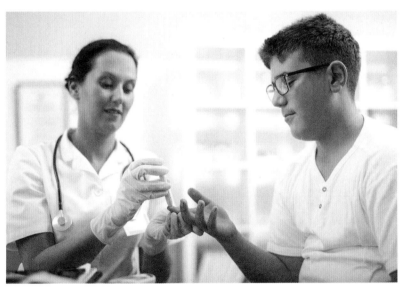

As a person with T1D, you are going to have a few different doctors throughout your life. You will most likely have a primary care doctor, someone you see once a year for an annual checkup or someone to approach if you need help when you are sick or hurt (not an emergency). You will also definitely have an **endocrinologist**, which is a fancy word for a diabetes doctor. In this chapter, I will talk briefly about your primary care doctor and more extensively about your diabetes doctor.

YOUR PRIMARY CARE DOCTOR

The main thing to know about your primary care doctor is that you and your parents have to keep him or her informed about your T1D. This can be easily done by making sure all the records your diabetes doctors have are released to your primary care doctor. Unlike your diabetes doctor, your primary care doctor takes care of your general health, so he or she needs to be aware of any and all health problems you are having. Having said this, remember that your general doctor is not your diabetes doctor. They may not be able to answer specific questions about your T1D as they are not T1D specialists; that is why you have a separate diabetes doctor. Do not get frustrated if your general doctor cannot answer your questions about T1D. You can ask if you would like, but make sure you also ask your diabetes doctors—they are the experts.

YOUR DIABETES DOCTOR

Going to your diabetes doctor can be overwhelming, especially the first few times. You may not know what questions to ask and may be unfamiliar with some of the terms they use. In this section, I will make going to your diabetes doctor easy by:

A. Defining some common diabetes terms used
B. Explaining what the various tests performed on you mean
C. Providing some helpful questions you might want to ask during an appointment

Terms and Tests

We have already talked about terms like *pancreas, insulin, carbohydrate, ketones* and *diabetic ketoacidosis (DKA)*, and *honeymoon phase*, but let's talk about a few others that might be new to you:

Basal Rate: I talked about this term in chapter 4, "Insulin on All Fronts: Injections and Pumps," but I would like to reiterate it here. This term is used a lot for people with insulin pumps. A basal rate is basically a steady amount of insulin that you receive to maintain your blood sugar. If you are not on a pump, the insulins Levemir or Lantus act as the "basal rate" in your insulin system. Basal rates differ from person to person, just like every factor of T1D.

Bolus: A bolus is just a bunch of insulin given at one time. The word is typically used when you give yourself a lot of insulin before a main meal. For example, when I eat my breakfast consisting of a massive bowl of cereal and whole milk, I will bolus by giving myself eight units of insulin (my bowl of cereal and milk is about eighty carbs, and I give myself one unit of insulin for every ten carbs I eat).

Terms can be kind of hard to understand until someone else breaks them down for you. The same can be said for tests that the diabetes doctors run. I always had trouble figuring out what each different test was, and many times when I received a test result, I would have no idea what the numbers meant. Here are explanations for some tests your diabetes doctors will run on you:

HbA1c: This is one of the most common tests that diabetes doctors will run on people with T1D. It is done every appointment and is basically an indicator of how well you are taking care of your T1D. Your diabetes doctors will tell you that any number under 7.0 is within the target range, and anything above 7.0 is outside the target range. *But what do these numbers even mean?* Your HbA1c level is defined as the amount of sugar that is covering your red blood cells, and in the US this is measured in a percentage. An HbA1c level of 7.0 actually means that your red blood cells are covered, on average, 7.0 percent by sugar. This makes complete sense because if you are not taking care of your T1D and are having a lot of high blood sugars, your red blood cells will be more covered (or saturated) in sugar, and therefore your HbA1c level will be higher. Doctors also say that this test is a good indication of how you have been taking care of your T1D for the last three months. *Why three months?* As it turns out, the average life of a red blood cell is three months. Thus, the HbA1c test is accurate up to the oldest red blood cells in your body, which are likely around three months old.

Regular Blood Drawings and *Urine Samples*: Before I got diagnosed with T1D, I hated getting my blood drawn. I did not do it a lot, but I never enjoyed the experience of having someone take blood out of a vein in my arm with a big needle. However, when I got T1D and had to get my blood drawn every six to twelve months or so, I got over it pretty quickly. To be honest, it is not that bad. It hurts for a half second when the person puts the needle into your arm, and that's it. No big deal. As a person with T1D, you will have to get your blood drawn pretty frequently, and a bunch of tests are run on your blood sample. *But what kind of tests?* A lot of people do not know this, but T1D is an **autoimmune disease**. This simply means that your body attacks itself. As I discussed earlier in this book, your body attacks the beta cells in your pancreas, which are the cells that produce insulin. Because T1D is an autoimmune disease, you have to keep a close eye on your body in case other parts of your body start malfunctioning and cause health issues, like thyroid disorders (problems with a gland in your neck) and celiac disease (autoimmune response to gluten that can cause harm to your small intestines). Blood tests are usually accompanied by urine samples too, which are used to make sure your kidneys are working properly. These regular blood tests and urine samples keep your doctors informed on how the rest of your body is doing and if anything is possibly being affected by your T1D.

Vision Tests and Circulation Tests: These tests may not arise until years after you have been diagnosed with T1D. They are conducted just to make sure that other parts of your body are not being harmed by your T1D. If you have too many high blood sugars for a very, very long time, they can end up negatively affecting parts of your body, such as your fingers, toes, and eyes. That is why vision and circulation tests are common every couple of years if you have had T1D for many years. If you take proper care of yourself, however, you should not have to worry about the results of these tests until you are older.

For a complete list of terms I mention throughout this book and their definitions, refer to the glossary on page 149.

Questions for the Diabetes Doctors

We have gone over different terms and tests your diabetes doctors might throw at you, but now it is time for you to toss questions back at them. Before I list some example questions, take note that if any of these terms or tests I mentioned above still do not make sense to you, feel free to ask your diabetes doctor. Always remember that your doctor is here to help you. Here are a few questions I have asked my diabetes doctors over the course of countless appointments:

- Do you think I am on the best plan to control my T1D? (pump vs. injection)
- Do you think I will eventually have to switch to a new system? When?
- Where is a good place to dispose of all my used needles?
- Can you examine my body to make sure I do not have any hard tissue spots from injecting insulin?
- What kind of technology has been coming out lately in the T1D industry?
- Have there been any recent breakthroughs in studies or research?
- How do I set up a 504 Plan? (I will talk about this in chapter 8, "Surviving School with T1D.")
- Where can I get a medical bracelet? (See the paragraph on medical bracelets below.)

Being Confident and Comfortable

In addition to asking helpful questions, there are a couple of other things you should make sure you and your parents have done so you can go into your appointments feeling confident and comfortable.

My first tip for both you and your parents: Before you leave your house, check to see if you need any prescription refills. Seeing your diabetes doctor is always a good time to get new prescriptions for ones that are going to expire soon or have already expired. Also, many diabetes doctors have tons of samples in their back closets. If you are unhappy with a certain BG meter or needle, check to see what your insurance covers and ask if you can try another type that is covered. I personally went through a bunch of different BG meter samples until I finally fell in love with the FreeStyle BG meter. Similarly, many diabetes doctors have various insulin pump models you can look at too. Again, checking with your insurance to see what pumps are covered is a good first step. While you cannot take them home with you, seeing the different pump models in person might help you make a decision if you're having trouble deciding on a pump you want to try. You should also consider specific pump features you are looking for, such as whether it is waterproof, has a remote control, or is compatible with CGM, and how much insulin it holds.

The next tip is kind of obvious and relates to any medical appointment: get to your doctor's office early. Even if you get there early and the doctor cannot see you until later, they can at least check you in and get some of the preliminary stuff done, such as measuring height, weight, blood pressure, and HbA1c level. Remember that you will have some visits where you only have a few issues to discuss, but on other visits you might have major issues that need to be addressed; the latter will therefore take more time. This, combined with how long other patients before you take, can greatly impact the flow of the doctor's office that day. What is most important is that you get the most out of your time with your clinician and understand that if he or she is running late, it is likely because another patient is having major struggles that day. Don't get frustrated if the wait is longer than expected (I still have trouble with this sometimes). Sit back, read a magazine, watch TV, play a game on your iPhone, and relax.

My next tip is related to comfort: wear comfortable clothes. This is another standard piece advice with any doctor's office, but it especially applies when going to your diabetes doctor. You always have to take your shoes off to get your height and roll up a sleeve to get your blood pressure. When your doctors check for hard tissue spots around your body, it is always easier when you have flexible clothes that allow easy access to your arms, legs, stomach, and any other places where you inject insulin or have pump sites.

MEDICAL BRACELET/NECKLACE/TATTOO

This topic is commonly overlooked but could save your life one day. I delayed getting a medical necklace for a while, but now I have one and never take it off. Your diabetes doctor can help you find a place that will make you a general or custom medical bracelet or necklace. You can also buy one online, at a jewelry store, or at any pharmacy. I got mine through a local jeweler where I could get it engraved. When choosing what to engrave on your necklace or bracelet, the three things I would put are first and last name, a telephone number to notify someone if you are hurt or sick (either your home phone number or one of your parents' cell phone numbers), and the statement "Type 1 Diabetes on insulin." The medical alert symbol with the snake wrapped around a pole is very recognizable, but it does not tell anyone why exactly you are wearing it; the statement "Type 1 Diabetes on insulin" clearly spells that out. I currently have these three things on my medical necklace. Similarly, you can also get a tattoo of this information somewhere on your body. The most common places people get a medical tattoo are usually somewhere on their wrist or forearm (where it is easy to spot by someone else, especially medical professionals).

The choice between a necklace, bracelet, or tattoo is purely personal, and one is not better than the other. A bracelet won't look out of place, but it is visible to others. A necklace, on the other hand, can be hidden under most shirts. A tattoo cannot really be hidden if it is on your arm or wrist and if you are wearing a short-sleeved shirt or dress, but you never have to worry about it falling off or getting lost. A couple of my friends, Nick and Allison, who are EMTs, say that a medical bracelet is easier to recognize because it is not usually covered by clothing, but both will do the job just fine. Choose whichever one you feel most comfortable wearing. After you have it on for a week or so, you will forget it is even there. For me, it has come to the point that whenever I am not wearing my medical necklace, I feel really weird and naked.

1

TELLING PEOPLE YOU KNOW

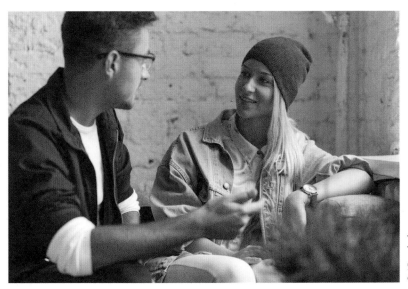

Having T1D can be stressful (I think we have all figured this out by now). And sometimes, you just want to handle it on your own. You feel like you are the only one who can understand and manage the pressure of T1D. I am very independent when it comes to my T1D, and sometimes that is an acceptable mindset to have. However, just as you have the responsibility to test your own blood sugar and give yourself insulin, you also have the responsibility of informing the people around you of your condition. Just because your T1D is *your* concern does not mean you should keep everyone else in the dark. Of course, your close family and loved ones all know you have T1D. They also should know how to handle certain situations if they arise, for example if you go low and cannot get yourself a glass of orange juice. Your family generally knows what you go through on a daily basis; however, you also go to school and interact with your teachers, coaches, classmates, and friends, all of whom need to know about your T1D too.

One of the most important things about being responsible and taking care of your T1D is making sure the people you surround yourself with know what you are experiencing. You do not have to tell everyone each little detail about how you manage your T1D, but telling key people some basics is necessary. You never know when your blood sugar might spike or drop and you might need help from a friend, teacher, or coach. People knowing that you have T1D will also help you in countless situations throughout life, including times when you have to temporarily leave class during school to test your blood sugar or when you need to take a break during soccer practice to get some sugar in your body. On top of that, telling people you have T1D allows you to create a reliable support system in the event that you fall into the all-too-common trap of "**diabetes burnout**," which basically refers to when people with T1D begin to neglect managing their T1D (because we just get so fed up and annoyed with it). The reasons *why* you should tell people you have T1D may be clear, but everything else might not seem so simple. In this chapter, I will go over who you should tell, what you should tell them, and how you should tell them.

WHO SHOULD YOU TELL?

Besides your immediate family, there are a few other people in your everyday life that should probably know you have T1D:

friends   teammates
romantic partners   coaches
neighbors   bosses
babysitters   coworkers
teachers

These are suggestions. If there are others you think you should add to the list, tell them as well. As the saying goes, "Better to be safe than sorry." It is a good idea to inform those closest to you that you have T1D.

WHAT SHOULD I TELL THEM?

Knowing *who* to tell is very important, but you have to know *what* to tell them as well. Here are some of the main points I discuss with people when I tell them I have T1D:

- *I have type 1 diabetes*: This is a pretty important one. Also reassure them that you know how to manage it. It will make them feel a lot more comfortable knowing you have a grip on the situation.
- Explain what T1D is: an autoimmune condition in which my body is unable to make insulin. Insulin is needed by the body to take up sugar and use it as fuel. Without insulin I can get sick, but otherwise I can do everything that other kids can do. (Also, T1D is not contagious.)
- I am on injections *or* I am on a pump.
- I wear a medical bracelet or necklace.
- I might have to excuse myself at some point to check/correct my blood sugar (this is important to tell teachers, bosses, coaches, etc.).
- If I happen to lose consciousness (which is unlikely to ever happen), I have an emergency glucagon kit here (name the location you keep it at). The directions are inside the kit and there is also a free phone application called "Glucagon"

that provides instructions on how to use it. Also, you should definitely call 911 if I lose consciousness.

• I would appreciate it if you could keep the fact that I have T1D to yourself, *or*, you can feel free to tell anyone I have T1D.

• Do you have any questions for me about T1D or how I manage it?

Again, this list is just a basic guideline, so if you think you should add anything that is not on this list, go ahead. A lot of times, people will ask questions about your T1D after you have finished explaining the basics. They may even share some stories and experiences they have had with other people with T1D.

HOW SHOULD YOU TELL THEM?

So far, we have gone over the easy stuff—who to tell and what to tell them. Those are just facts. You can make a checklist (like I did above) and hit each one of the bullet points one at a time. This next section is not as easy. We may know we have to tell someone, and what to tell him or her, but we could have trouble actually doing it. I have always been a fairly outgoing person, but even I have struggled with finding the best way to tell someone I have T1D. Here, I will share the easiest ways I have found to inform someone about my T1D.

This first part might sound obvious, but when telling people you have T1D, do not dance around the subject. Tell it to them straight. The worst thing you can do is drag on a conversation and not get to your point; eventually, even you will forget what you wanted to tell them. You just have to say it. Rip it off like a bandage.

Another tip I can give is that the first time you plan to tell someone, try to do it in person. You can definitely continue the discussion about your T1D in greater detail over the phone or by text or email, but the first time should really be in person, if possible. I have found that it is usually easier to communicate when you are looking someone in the face. It can be hard facing another person, but trust me, the entire conversation will go much more smoothly.

It also gives the person you are informing a chance to directly ask you any questions they might have.

If you need to tell a certain person you have T1D but are in the middle of a bunch of people who, for whatever reason, you do not want to know you have T1D, it is perfectly okay to pull that person aside and talk privately. At the very least, go up to that person and make it clear you want to chat: "Hey, I have to talk to you about something later. Nothing bad, I just have to tell you something. When would be a good time to chat?" At least at this point the person is aware you have to tell them something. If you want to tell one of your teachers and you do not want other students in your class to know, wait until class is dismissed. The same can be said if you are at work and need to tell your boss but do not want your coworkers knowing. Some of my friends who have T1D choose to tell certain people and exclude others. I, however, see very little harm in telling anyone and everyone around you.

Letting someone know that you have T1D helps both you and the person you are telling; it makes that person feel prepared and makes you feel safe. You do not want to put someone in a position of helplessness if anything happens to you and they have absolutely no idea what to do. How would you feel if your friend who has T1D did not tell you about their medical situation, and when they had a low blood sugar episode you had no idea what was going on? This is how I judge any given situation: What would I want someone to do if I was on the other side of the information? Additionally, now that you have told that person, you can feel confident knowing that if something goes wrong, there will be someone who can help you.

Remember, too, that this does not have to be a big formal occasion. You do not have to go out to lunch with someone just to tell them that you have T1D. It can be as simple as letting someone know when you pass them in a hallway. Everything you need to convey can be said in less than two minutes. Take your time, pick the right moment, and do not shy away from anything you think they need to hear. This is for both you and the person you are telling. At this point in my life, I basically tell all the people who play a role in my life that I have T1D. I tell them in a matter-of-fact manner, like I would about any other piece of trivial information about myself: "Hi, my name is Patrick, I am twenty-two, I love the New York Giants, and I have T1D."

8

SURVIVING SCHOOL WITH T1D

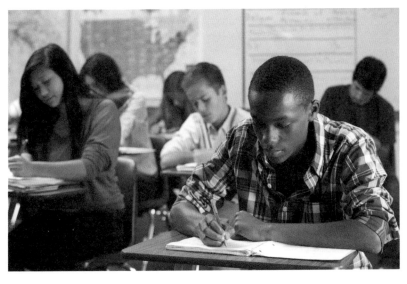

© iStockphoto

Having already gone through elementary school, middle school, high school, and most of college, I can confirm that school is not always easy. All academic settings come with their own obstacles: homework, quizzes, tests, projects . . . and those are just school related. There are also plenty of other distractions that can affect your everyday life while in school: sports, clubs, and friends, just to name a few. School is daunting enough as it is, and now you have to add T1D to the pile . . . yippee! This chapter is meant to be your personal guide as you navigate school with T1D. I will touch on all the major topics and scenarios I have experienced while walking through the halls during my time as a student.

SCHEDULES

Regardless of grade or institution, every student at school follows a schedule. Some people have math class in the morning and PE in the afternoon, while others have a rotating schedule that puts classes at different times each day. In any case, your school schedule will actually help you control your T1D. Schedules are always good for people with T1D because it gives us strict and constant times within our days to take care of our blood sugar. For me, it was a relief to know that I would have lunch at eleven thirty every morning. I always knew when I would test my blood sugar and take my insulin.

When you get into high school, there are opportunities for "free periods"—some call these periods "enrichment" while others call them "study hall." Despite the different names, these periods are also great times to test your blood sugar and make sure it is where it is supposed to be. Having said this, I never shy away from testing my blood sugar in class if I feel I need to. If you feel a low blood sugar coming on, you would be putting your health in danger if you did not test as soon as possible (I will talk about how to approach testing your blood sugar in class a little later in this chapter).

HEALTH/NURSE'S OFFICE

I have never been to a school that did not have a health office. Where there are people, there is sickness, and where there is sickness, there is a place for the sick to go. One of the first things I do every year of school is go into the health office and talk with one of the nurses, even if it is just to say, "Hello, my name is Patrick McAllister and I have T1D. Goodbye." It is better than making no contact whatsoever. On top of going in and saying hello, I also always give the nurses extra supplies at the beginning of every school year to keep in the office in case I need something in a pinch:

- emergency glucagon kit
- instant glucose gel
- test strips
- extra BG meter (in case mine dies)
- a sixteen-pack of juice boxes *or* a fifty-pack of glucose tablets
- insulin—whatever kinds you might need while at school (if you are on a pump, you may need to bring extra rapid-acting and long-acting insulin in case the pump fails while at school)
- insulin pump sites and/or CGM sites
- AAA batteries for your pump or continuous glucose monitor (CGM)

These supplies may seem like overkill, but trust me, keeping extra supplies in a place you frequent eight hours a day, five days a week is a really safe idea and can prevent you from having to miss school. Like I always say, it is better to be safe than sorry. Another good tip is to make sure you put your name on all your supplies—you can do what I do and throw it all in a big Ziploc bag with your name written on the outside. You might not be the only person with T1D at your school, and the last thing you want is your supplies getting mixed up with someone else's. Also, a precaution to take is to check the expiration dates on all your supplies at the end of each semester. Make sure nothing has expired or gone bad. It is also a good idea to keep extra supplies in your sports bag or with you for extracurricular activities after the nurse's office is closed.

If you are one of those people who really does not enjoy going to your nurse's office, then do not feel pressured to frequent it if you do not have to. After I was diagnosed in middle school, I was required to go to my nurse's office before lunch every day to test my blood sugar. I actually enjoyed this routine. Just know that you are not alone if you are on one of these strict regimens. However, the nurse's office can be a very valuable resource at school. It's an excellent safe haven if you ever want to test and correct your blood sugar levels. You are free from all pressures that might be lurking in the classroom: no one looking at you while you test your blood sugar, no one asking if they can have one of your glucose tablets, and no feeling of panic that you are not paying attention to the information on the board. In the nurse's office, it is just you and the nurses. In middle school and high school, I found it very comforting to have a stress-free place to go whenever I needed to test my blood sugar. On top of that, the nurses at my middle school were some of the nicest individuals I have ever met. No matter the school, every nurse I have dealt with has been extremely friendly and accommodating.

Essentially, the frequency with which you go to your nurse's office is a joint decision between you, your family, the nurse, and your diabetes doctor. If the decision is left up to you, do not feel pressured to stop by every week, but also do not feel like you are burdening the nurses if you go in every day. Their job is to help you take care of your health, and they should be happy to help take care of you.

TELLING TEACHERS

In addition to actually teaching you, teachers provide a multitude of other services at any given school. Many teachers are advisors to different clubs, some are coaches of school sports teams, and some will even bring in cookies or cupcakes when it is someone's birthday. I like to think of teachers as your parents when you are at school. And just as your real parents care that your T1D is under control, so do your teachers. Teachers not only want you to learn the material that is in their classes; they also want you to be healthy and safe. For this reason, it is a *must* that you inform all your teachers you have T1D.

In chapter 7, "Telling People You Know," I discussed the need to inform your friends about your T1D—if the time comes when you are unable to correct a low or high blood sugar, they will be able to help you. Your teachers must be informed for the same reason. They are the most likely candidates to actually help you if anything goes wrong while in school, and they need to know the main points of your T1D. It can be kind of awkward trying to find a time and place to tell your teachers; I either waited until after class or went in early in the morning before school started. It is always good to get this done as soon as possible. Do not wait until school starts to inform your teachers; try to get into contact or meet with them as soon as you can. In high school, my guidance counselor set up a meeting at the beginning of every school year with my teachers, my parents, and me in order to make sure everyone was on the same page about my T1D. For any other tips on what to tell your teachers and how to tell them, refer to chapter 7, "Telling People You Know."

504 PLAN

I had no idea what a 504 Plan was before I was diagnosed with T1D, but I now realize how helpful it can be. A 504 Plan is a legal document that recognizes you as an individual with a legitimate disability and outlines reasonable accommodations that can prevent T1D from getting in the way of your learning and help you succeed at school. Put simply, it is a document that lays out a plan for how your school can help you with your T1D. This includes but is not limited to:

- testing and correcting your blood sugar in class;
- leaving class to test and correct your blood sugar (even during a quiz or test);
- receiving makeup time on a quiz or test if you have to leave to correct your blood sugar; and
- receiving extra time and/or private proctoring on standardized tests so you can stop and test/correct your blood sugars without being penalized if the standardized test is timed (like the SAT or ACT).

This document is also a support system for you if any of these accommodations are not being met. I have never had this happen to me, but my older cousin, Casey, had a teacher in high school who did not let her make up time on a test that she had to leave in the middle of to correct a low blood sugar. She had a 504 Plan, and when she brought the scenario to her parents' attention, they told the principal, and everything was straightened out.

As I have mentioned, at the start of every school year in high school, my parents and I met with all my teachers, as well as my guidance counselor and principal, to go over my 504 Plan and make sure everyone was on the same page. In addition, when I took my SAT and ACT during my junior and senior years of high school, I was separated from the rest of the students and given a private proctor who would stop the timer if I needed to test my blood sugar. I didn't like this accommodation at first because I didn't want to be separated from everyone else, but looking back, being by myself was great. Speaking as a student, I found it much easier to concentrate while taking the tests alone in an absolutely silent room.

At times, the 504 Plan may feel like you are cheating the system: *Why am I allowed extra time on a test? Why am I allowed to leave the classroom without even asking?* You need to understand that you are not cheating in the slightest, and that this legal document is put in place in order to help you. Your peers might tease you because of the accommodations you receive, but they do not know what you are experiencing, so do not let it bother you. It is better to have a 504 Plan and never use it than not to have a 504 Plan and need it when a person or situation at school treats you unfairly because of your T1D. You do not have to use the accommodations listed if you do not want to, but having them in place will help you in case any situation arises that attempts to punish you because of your T1D. Talk with your diabetes doctor and your school guidance counselor or advisor to get an individualized 504 Plan up and running. If you want to look at some models of 504 Plan formats or have any more questions with regards to 504 Plans, the American Diabetes Association has a very helpful and accessible page on their website (www.diabetes.org: go to "Living With Diabetes," then "For Parents & Kids," then "Safe at School," and then finally "Written Care Plans").

CHECKING AND CORRECTING YOUR BLOOD SUGAR

Just because you are at school does not mean you are exempt from checking your blood sugar and taking care of yourself. In fact, it is quite the opposite. You need to be at your very best when you are at school so you can learn and do your very best on all of your exams. Therefore, it is crucial to make sure your T1D is kept under control at all times. However, I understand that it can be hard sometimes to check and correct your blood sugar right in the middle of a math lesson or a Spanish quiz. You have to remember that your T1D is not just a challenge you live with; it is an important aspect of your life. No matter where you are or what you do, your health and well-being should always come first. There are different ways to approach testing and correcting your blood sugar in the classroom, and I will give you some pointers based on how I went about testing and correcting my blood sugar throughout middle and high school. If I ever felt low or high, I would do one of two things:

1. **Test and correct my blood sugar at my seat.** I did this for most of my classes. Thankfully, testing your blood sugar only takes thirty seconds or so and is therefore not a huge distraction to the rest of the class.
2. **Politely excuse myself and walk to the nurse's office to test and correct my blood sugar.** If I really felt uncomfortable testing and correcting my blood sugar in class, or I felt that correcting my blood sugar was going to require special attention, I would simply tell my teacher, "I am headed to the nurse's office." I have *never* received any kind of backlash from teachers when I informed them I needed to excuse myself to take care of my T1D. On the contrary, I would often be

asked if I wanted someone to escort me to the nurse's office (my friends loved this because it got them out of class for a couple of minutes). So, if you ever feel really low or high and need someone to walk with you to the nurse's office, just ask. It is better to ask than to end up passing out in the hallway from a low blood sugar.

ACING QUIZZES AND TESTS

Taking quizzes and tests are part of school; it's just the way it goes. You are supposed to be learning information throughout your school years, and tests are a way of checking to see if you have retained that information. Two of the main factors that accompany tests are stress and nervousness. Even after my ten years of experience taking tests, I still get nervous before every single one. The test-taking environment can really send your blood sugar levels on a ride, and the ride can be different for everyone. Some of my friends always get high blood sugars from taking tests, while I have gotten both low and high blood sugars. In this section, I will tell you what I do to prepare for every test and quiz I take.

First, I make sure I eat a good breakfast (or lunch, if the test is in the afternoon). For me, this normally consists of a bowl of healthy cereal—not Lucky Charms or Reese's Puffs—coupled with a banana. Having food in your system is extremely important to doing well on exams. Your brain needs energy to think, and if you do not supply it with enough food to turn into energy, it is not going to function at its very best. Second, I make sure I bring my BG meter, insulin, and a source of sugar to my test. You should always have these things with you anyway, but I like to double-check to make sure I am fully prepared for my exam.

After I enter the room, the first thing I do after getting my pencils and paper out is test my blood sugar. Do this as soon as you get settled. Give yourself a time cushion in case you need to make any kind of blood sugar corrections before your test begins. If I test my blood sugar and am in the sweet spot (target range), I still make sure I have a source of sugar out of my backpack and within reach. I do not want to have to search for my glucose tablets in the middle of a test if I feel my blood sugar starting to drop.

During the test, if I feel my blood sugar start to rise or fall, I assess the situation and determine if I can continue to take the test. If the symptoms are relatively moderate and I can easily correct my blood sugar, I do so. If, on the other hand, I do not think that I can finish the test or that it is going to take more than ten minutes to fully correct my blood sugar, I walk up to my teacher, inform them about my situation, and head to the nurse's office. I did this once for a Spanish exam. At the end of the day, I went back and told my teacher I was sorry I had to leave in the middle of her exam, at which point she actually got a little mad at me—not because I left early but because I had apologized. She then proceeded to ask me about fifteen times if I was okay and then allowed me to finish the test the next day after school. Your 504 Plan ensures that this option is available to you, but I highly doubt any teacher is going to give you problems. With the exception of a few bad eggs, all teachers want to see you succeed. If you have to leave a class to correct your blood sugar, your teacher will understand.

After I finish the exam and walk out of the room, I always test my blood sugar again to double-check and make sure nothing crazy happened while I was taking the test. In addition, if the test I am taking is a real whopper, for example a three- or four-hour Advanced Placement (AP) exam, after the test is over I keep a closer eye on my blood sugar for the next couple of hours. Sometimes the effects of taking an exam are a little delayed, and I do not want any surprises. If you follow these steps when taking a test or quiz, I have no doubt you will perform your very best on every single one (provided you actually study for it).

LUNCH AND THE CAFETERIA

Since you are at school for roughly eight hours a day, you are going to need to eat. Every school has a cafeteria a time period to eat. These strict time periods are great because they provide you with structured and unchanging intervals to test your blood sugar, inject insulin, and eat. I found it relatively easy to remember to test and take insulin once I got into a routine at school, but I know one of my friends with T1D sets an alarm to remind himself. Regardless of if you bring your own lunch from home or buy lunch at school, be mindful of when you give yourself insulin and how much you give. I was able to wait until I sat down to take my insulin for lunch, but some people need to take insulin fifteen minutes before eating in order to prevent high blood sugar. If you usually take insulin a little while before you eat, my advice is to take a small dose of insulin in your class before lunch or before getting in line at the cafeteria. Take the rest just before starting to eat. This should help prevent super high or low blood sugar levels following lunch. I usually brought in my own lunch, but once in middle school I had to buy lunch from the cafeteria, and I decided to take all my insulin before getting into the lunch line. The lunch line was extremely long and slow that day, and by the time I finally got my food I had to take some glucose tablets to correct the low blood sugar caused by the insulin I had injected prematurely. You never know how long the lunch line is going to be and how fast it is going to move, so play it safe and wait until you sit down at the table to take your insulin.

Additionally, many cafeterias offer a variety of snacks you can buy. Definitely feel free to get some, but make sure you know what you are eating. Some snacks, such as Fruit Snacks and Doritos, will have the nutritional label on the bag. Other snacks, however, like nachos with cheese and hot pretzels, might be handed out without any sort of packaging. Make sure you know how many carbs you are putting into your system. If you have already taken insulin for your lunch carbs but then decide you really want that hot pretzel, make sure you take more insulin to cover those extra carbs. Do not brush it off and say, "Well, it's okay. It's only a couple extra carbs, and I already took my insulin." Do not be ignorant of your body's needs, and remember to take insulin for any significant number of carbs you eat or drink.

You might have questions about the food you are buying: *How many carbs are in this? Has any extra sugar been added to that?* The best thing to do in this case is to ask one of the cafeteria workers. Many times, they should be able to answer your questions almost immediately. At the very least, they should be able to find the cafeteria manager, who will be able to answer your questions.

A common scenario I found myself in during school lunches was sitting with my friends and getting so caught up talking with them that I forgot to eat all of my lunch. Sometimes I took insulin for sixty carbs and only ate thirty carbs. In this case, it is okay to bring the rest of your lunch with you to your next class and finish eating it there. Every school has a slightly different policy around eating during class, but you should be able to work out an acceptable plan with your school nurse and teachers that allows you to eat/finish your lunch during class if necessary. Do not throw your lunch away and leave your body with an excess amount of insulin; if you do this you *will* get low blood sugar, and you *will* have to stop working or even possibly leave class in order to correct your blood sugar. I have done this before, and it is not fun. Try really hard to eat as many carbs as you gave yourself insulin for. You can also talk to your doctor if your carb targets for meals seem too high or low so your plan can be adjusted.

GYM CLASS

Whether you are an athlete or not, everyone who goes to school is required to take gym class or, as most schools call it nowadays, physical education (PE). Gym class is meant to give students a break from the normal classroom setting and get them physically active. Although gym class is not nearly as intense as an organized sports team, since you are participating in a physical activity, you have to watch out for your blood sugar.

After changing into my gym clothes and just before gym class started, I would sit down and quickly test my blood sugar to make sure it was okay to be active for an entire class period. When I was diagnosed with T1D in middle school, all of my friends were very supportive, and one of them in particular, Jack, wanted to learn how to test my blood sugar. I showed him one day in the locker room before gym class, and from that day on, he named himself my personal nurse. Before every gym class, I would give him my BG meter kit, and he would set everything up for me. Not bad, right? I paid him in glucose tablets, which he seemed to think was a fair trade-off for thirty seconds of BG-meter prep.

The last thing I will say about taking care of your T1D during gym class is to be aware of the intensity of the physical activities that day before you do anything drastic, like drinking a juice to raise your blood sugar or lowering your insulin in preparation for an anticipated low blood sugar. If you are running a mile or playing an intense game of dodgeball, feel free to take the necessary precautions to prevent a low blood sugar. However, if you are going to be participating in something that requires significantly less energy, like juggling, you might want to rethink how much you alter your normal T1D management routine.

FIELD TRIPS

Ironically, some of the most fun times during school are field trips (when you're not actually at school). Field trips are great breaks from regular schoolwork, and, if you are lucky, you will get to see some pretty cool stuff too. I remember two of my particularly favorite field trips: Ellis Island during middle school and Universal Studios in Florida during high school with the concert band. Field trips are really special experiences, and the last thing you want to do is ruin your experience because your T1D is giving you trouble.

First, get information about the specifics. Here are a few questions you need to be able to answer before venturing on a field trip:

- Where are we going?
- How long are we going for?

- Will we be on the field trip during a mealtime?
- Will there be food provided or are we expected to bring our own food?

The answers to these questions will help you plan how to approach the field trip. The next step is to pack what you need. Regardless of place or duration, you should always bring the following:

- BG meter (with plenty of test strips)
- Insulin (for daily injections or pump) and extra pump sites (in case the one you have on expires or falls off)
- Extra sensor with inserter if you use a continuous glucose monitor (CGM)
- Supply of sugar (juice or glucose tablets)
- A couple of dollars for soda or juice (just in case you need sugar or food and it is being sold around you)
- Instant glucose gel and emergency glucagon kit (and someone who knows how to use it)
- Some kind of identification that you have T1D (usually in the form of a note from your diabetes doctor, which you can request at any time; this is particularly helpful if you need to get your backpack full of supplies into a place that does not normally allow backpacks, like museums)
- Medical alert bracelet

Since you are going on a school field trip, you will most likely already be bringing your backpack, which you can use to store these supplies. Depending on where you are going and for how long, you might need to modify some of the items listed above. For example, if you take multiple kinds of insulin for your daily injections routine and are staying overnight somewhere, you will have to pack those extra types of insulin for breakfast the following morning. Likewise, if you are going to be away for an extended amount of time, like my trip to Universal Studios in Florida, you might have to pack extra test strips, pump sites, and even BG meter batteries. In addition, if you know you are supposed to provide your own food during the field trip, pack accordingly to make sure you have enough food to last however long you will be on the trip (or bring money to buy food). If the trip includes air travel, always keep your T1D supplies in your carry-on (I discuss how to travel on airplanes with T1D in chapter 10, "Traveling with T1D").

The last important note is to inform your teacher or chaperone of your T1D. I hope I have driven this lesson into your head by now—it is crucial to let the people around you know that you have T1D, especially the people responsible for your health and safety. In some cases, your teachers or chaperones will want to hold on to your emergency glucagon kit so they have it if it needs to be used. If you keep supplies in your nurse's office at school, which I mentioned earlier in this chapter, you can ask them to pack the supplies for you. When I was in middle school, whenever I went on a field trip, the school nurses would pack my supplies in a large medical bag for the teacher or chaperone and then put them back when the field trip was over. You might not get as lucky as me, but be mindful that the supplies in your nurse's office are at your disposal for use on field trips.

9

HERE'S THE GAME PLAN — TID AND SPORTS

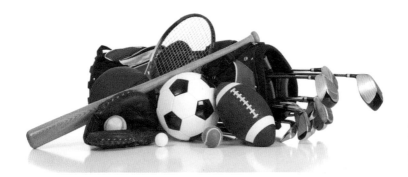

I have been playing sports for as long as I can remember. I love the healthy competition and constant physical and mental action that surrounds every sport. When I was diagnosed with T1D, I knew that being physically active was definitely going to come with its fair share of challenges, but it in no way discouraged me from playing sports. Throughout this chapter, I will discuss how to manage your T1D when playing sports or working out in general, and then I will explore how to handle specific sports. My greatest piece of advice to you is never to let your T1D get in the way of being physically active. It might be difficult, even annoying at times, but you can do it. If I decided to cut myself off from sports when I was diagnosed with T1D, I would have lost a part of my life that was very important to me. Fortunately, I figured out how to be an athlete with T1D, and you can too.

Whenever you participate in a sport, you are physically active. Whether it is basketball, baseball, or bowling, you are exerting physical energy in some capacity. Because of this, your body is using up more sugar than usual to provide energy to your body as you move. As a result, you are more prone to have low blood sugars. This means that you have to pay very close attention to make sure your blood sugar levels do not plummet while you are active.

Additionally, the majority of the sports you might participate in will take place outside on a hot, sunny day or inside in a similarly hot court. Even if you are skiing on a cold winter day, you are probably wrapped up in many layers of clothing, which is going to make the immediate area around your body very hot. Heat tends to cause your blood sugar levels to drop because it "superactivates" the insulin already in your body. This, combined with the fact that your body has to use more energy to stay at a normal temperature, can really tank your blood sugar. Know the environment you are playing in, and make sure to account for the heat that might make your blood sugar drop.

PREVENTATIVE MEASURES

A good way to prevent low blood sugars while playing sports or working out is to test before starting your activity. Before every soccer practice in middle school and high school, I would test my blood sugar to make sure I was in a comfortable range to be physically active. This range varies for each sport, and I will discuss specific sports later in this chapter. Generally, you want your blood sugar to be a little higher than normal when engaging in a sport. In chapter 3, "Those Darn Low and High Blood Sugars," I discussed that the sweet spot for your blood sugar is between 70 and 150. Before physical activity, however, you want your blood sugar generally between 150 and 200. This slight increase in your blood sugar range gives you a little cushion if (and when) your blood sugar starts to drop.

Another great way to prevent low blood sugars is to eat or drink something substantial before you start. It can be difficult sometimes to eat a lot before physical activity, but if you eat the right foods, they will help sustain your blood sugars over the period of time you are active. In chapter 2, "Carbohydrates—How to Eat and Drink with T1D," I talked about *complex carbs* and the fact that they last longer because they take a longer time for your body to break down. Here are a few of my personal favorite snacks to eat and drink before and while I am active, many of which contain complex carbs:

- *Bananas*: This is probably my favorite option for several reasons. On top of having a respectable number of carbs (twenty to twenty-five), bananas also contain lots of potassium, which is a great preventative for muscle cramping. Many of my teammates who do not have T1D would eat bananas prior to a big game.
- *Peanut butter*: If you have it on bread, the fat and protein in the peanut butter will help extend the carbs in the bread and sustain your blood sugar (I would almost ritualistically make myself a peanut butter and butter sandwich in preparation for practices and games—try it before you judge me).
- *Granola bars*: Granola bars, as opposed to solely nuts, are usually sweetened with a sugary ingredient, often raisins or chocolate. Granola bars are great because they are not too heavy and can be eaten rather quickly. I used to eat a granola bar during the halftimes of my soccer and lacrosse games.
- *Gatorade/water mix*: This is the smartest idea for T1D and sports! Instead of using just water to hydrate or Gatorade to correct your low blood sugars, combine the two into the

perfect low blood sugar-preventing drink. Make a fifty-fifty mix of water and Gatorade and sip on it throughout the duration of your sport. It might not always prevent a low blood sugar, but it will definitely slow the descent. When I played soccer and lacrosse, this mix stopped me from going low many times. It has a pretty dull taste, but its function completely outweighs its relative lack of flavor. (Note: I have noticed that the G2 Gatorade, which is manufactured with less sugar, does not have the same preventative effects as the fifty-fifty mix of water and regular Gatorade.)

The specifics of my next piece of advice will differ if you are on daily injections or an insulin pump. If you are on daily injections, it might be a good idea to lower your insulin doses before participating in a sport. I have done this for games and tournaments because these events are usually more intense and last longer than practices. Definitely talk with your diabetes doctor before changing anything, but know that it is an option to consider. If you use an insulin pump, you have a couple of options. Whenever my friend used to play soccer, he would simply detach his pump and cannula from his infusion site in order to stop the basal insulin drip he received. This is a great option to prevent you from going low, but make sure you remember to reattach your pump after you are finished. One of my teammates on my high school soccer team frequently forgot to put his pump back on after soccer practice and his blood sugar would be up in the 400s when dinnertime rolled around. An hour or so after you put your pump back on, test your blood sugar to make sure it is working. If you have a wireless pump, like I do, you may have the option of selecting "Suspend Insulin." I just input the duration I want my basal insulin intake to stop, and when that time is up, the pump will turn my basal dose back on.

Everything I have discussed so far relates to your blood sugar going low. This is because the majority of the problems people with T1D face when engaging in physical activity are low blood sugars.

However, it is also possible to have high blood sugars when playing sports. This usually happens after a sporting event is over. If you ate or drank a lot of carbs in an attempt to prevent a low blood sugar but did not use all of those carbs up, high blood sugar levels are a likely possibility. I remember playing a lacrosse game in which we were absolutely dominating the other team to the point that all of us starters were taken out after halftime. In preparation for the game, I had lowered my insulin and had a snack before we started, and I did not account for the decrease in playing time. A couple of hours after the game ended, my blood sugar was in the 300s. The best way to prevent this from happening is to make sure you test your blood sugar whenever you get a break. Also, do not forget to test thirty minutes or so after you have finished playing a sport to see how your blood sugar levels are doing.

CORRECTING LOWS AND HIGHS

You can do everything imaginable to stop a low or high blood sugar from coming on, but sometimes it still happens. With this in mind, you must learn how to correct low and high blood sugars during a sporting event. Let's start with low blood sugars.

The principle for correcting low blood sugars while playing sports is basically the same as it is when you normally correct with the "test and rest" method, with just a few additional nuances. The first specific is the number of carbs you use to correct your low. If you are playing a really intense sport, such as soccer, track, basketball, hockey, or lacrosse, you might want to correct with more than just the normal 16g of carbs. I would suggest correcting with between 20g and 30g instead. Another important factor you need to change when correcting a low blood sugar while active is the amount of time you rest while your blood sugar recovers. Even though you may stop and rest to test your blood sugar and drink a juice, your body is still consuming energy from the physical activity you were previously engaged in. Instead of waiting ten to fifteen minutes for your blood sugar to rise, I would wait at least twenty minutes.

After twenty minutes, you will have a better idea of whether your blood sugar is actually rebounding. And lastly, before getting up and going back out onto the field, court, track, rink, or wherever you are headed, make sure you test your blood sugar again. The only way you can be absolutely positive your blood sugar is actually recovering is to double-check.

Generally, high blood sugars are much easier than low blood sugars to correct when playing sports. This is because your body is constantly using energy while playing a sport, so if you ever happen to run into a high blood sugar, your body will already be actively helping you to lower it. Still, you should take extra caution when correcting a high blood sugar because it is hard to predict how much and how quickly your blood sugar will drop. Once, in the middle of a soccer practice, I tested my blood sugar and found myself in the 300s, so I took a little insulin to help bring it down. An hour later, however, I felt really terrible, and when I tested I was 83. Make sure you do not overshoot and give yourself too much insulin to correct a high blood sugar while playing a sport. Bring your correction factor ratio down to account for your physical activity. If your blood sugar is under 300, I would leave it alone; do not correct with insulin just yet. Drink some water, go back to playing your sport, and check again in twenty minutes. Odds are your blood sugar will naturally drop from the water, heat, and physical activity, so correcting with insulin would be overkill. The best thing you can do for correcting high blood sugars is to assess your situation. If you are playing a very active sport, you can probably bet that your blood sugar will drop on its own. However, if you are playing a less active sport, such as golf or bowling, you might want to think about taking a little insulin.

Managing T1D and sports is absolutely doable. However, it can also be unpredictable. Most of the time, your T1D will be a minor factor when being active, but it can creep up on you and really stop you in your tracks. The best thing you can do for your blood sugar and your body is to remain aware of how you are feeling (i.e., do you have symptoms of high or low blood sugar?). When in doubt, stop for a few seconds and test your blood sugar. This simple and proactive strategy has helped me to avoid the loss of countless playing hours over the course of my athletic career.

SPECIFIC SPORTS

Having provided a general overview of how to manage your T1D while being physically active, I will now give advice on how to manage your blood sugar when playing certain types of sports. Below, I have listed just a few examples of sports, ones I am at least somewhat familiar with. If you play a sport that is not listed, try comparing it to a sport I do discuss and that you think it is similar to. I have arranged the sports alphabetically.

Baseball/Softball: Since this is not the most intense sport in the world, it should be fairly easy to manage your blood sugar levels while playing. There is a lot of standing around, and you are in the dugout every half inning to watch your teammates bat (which can be a great time to test your blood sugar). Do not start your blood sugar much higher than 150 for games. You might want to start a little closer to 200 for practices, as those will probably be more physically intense than the games.

Basketball: The intensity of this sport can vary based on what position you play and how long your shifts are. Point guards naturally do more physical work than centers, but regardless, everyone is running up and down the court. Also, the sport is usually played inside on a hot and sticky court, which can cause your blood sugar levels to drop quickly. If you are a starter, your blood sugar should start around 200. If you are coming off the bench, you can start a little lower and take a swig of Gatorade before going into the game. The great thing about basketball is that there are a lot of timeouts that will provide you with opportunities to check and correct your blood sugar.

Cheerleading/Dancing: Dancing and cheerleading can take many forms, including competition formats, and require extreme amounts of physical and mental attention. It depends on what type of dancing you are doing, but you usually want to start your activity with your blood sugar a little below 200. At recitals, the musical numbers usually take five minutes or so, and you should be able to check your blood sugar after. Make sure you always have a source of sugar offstage that works quickly, such as glucose tablets or juice. For cheerleading, you should have no trouble finding time in between routines to check your blood sugar.

Cross Country: This can be an extremely difficult sport to manage your blood sugar during because you are running nonstop for a long time without any breaks. Make sure your blood sugar is a little over 200 before you start running. Whenever I run a 5K race, I keep a couple of glucose tablets in my pocket to chomp on throughout the race. I do not even test; I just pop them in my mouth as a preventative measure. This is one of the sports where you should definitely keep an eye on your blood sugar a few hours after the event is over, too, as your muscles will still be burning energy (using sugar) long after you have stopped running.

Fencing: While not as common as baseball or basketball, fencing is a growing sport—and I played it in high school, so I've included it here. There are tons of breaks during this sport, so you should be able to control your blood sugar in between matches with ease. Try to start your blood sugar between 175 and 200. However, since you work your legs so much during matches, you need to keep a special eye on your blood sugar for a couple hours after the match or tournament ends (like you would if you just ran a long distance run). I was astounded at the fact that I would frequently get a low blood sugar several hours after a tournament ended. You are also wearing a lot of gear, which can get really hot, so keep hydrated and watch for your blood sugar levels to drop.

Field Hockey and Lacrosse (Lax): While it depends on your position, you want to start your blood sugar a little below 200. If you are a goalie or play defense, keep a Gatorade in the net. Rotations happen quickly for middies in lax and field hockey (players who may play on both sides of the field), so you will have time to test and rest. If you are an attackman or defenseman, you will have time to rest when the ball is on the other side of the field. The other good thing is that there is substitution on the fly, so you can get in and out of the game much quicker than other sports, should you start to feel a low or high blood sugar. There are also a good number of timeouts in these sports, so you will have chances to check and correct then too.

Football: This is a sport that consists of a lot of short and intense plays. If you play on both sides of the ball, you should start your blood sugar around 200. The good thing is that if you only play on one side of the ball, you will have time to recover when the other side is on the field. Many times, a football team has a lot of players, so someone else can temporarily fill in for you if you need to check and correct your blood sugar.

Golf: Exertion for this sport can vary based on the weather conditions, as well as how many holes you are playing. Since you have plenty of walking time and can carry tons of supplies in your golf bag, I would suggest starting your blood sugar between 150 and 175. If it is really hot, make sure you check your blood sugar after every couple of holes (just don't let your BG meter beep right in the middle of someone else's backswing).

Ice Hockey: This is similar in style to lacrosse and field hockey because it consists of a lot of short, intense shifts with regulated breaks. Start your blood sugar somewhere around 200. If you are a goalie, keep a Gatorade in the net. Rotations happen quickly in hockey, so you will have time to test and rest. Like lacrosse, there is on-the-fly substituting as well, so you can easily remove yourself if you need to test and correct your blood sugar.

Lacrosse: See *Field Hockey*.

Skiing/Snowboarding: This is a sport and activity that can vary greatly with respect to energy expended. You could be riding on the slope with your friends or in serious downhill competition. If you tend to be more intense on the mountain, you should start your blood sugar around 200. If you are like me and are a fan of the laid-back joyrides down the slope, you can start your blood sugar a little lower, somewhere between 150 and 175. One of the good things about ski equipment is that your clothing usually has loads of pockets, so you should have plenty of space for your T1D supplies. On the other hand, you have to be extra careful with your BG meter and insulin because of the cold temperatures. I went skiing once for four hours, and when I went back into the lodge to eat lunch, I could not test my blood sugar because my BG meter said it was too cold to work. I had to remove and warm the batteries with my hands for five minutes before they were warm enough to function. Similarly, if your insulin gets too cold, it will not work properly. Keep your insulin and BG meter either in a pocket that you know will not get too cold or in a bag that will stay inside the ski lodge.

Soccer: This is one of the most difficult sports during which to maintain stable blood sugar levels because of the nonstop action. I played soccer all throughout middle school and high school and had my fair share of troubles. Start your blood sugar between 200 and 250 at the beginning of a practice or game. Remember to test your blood sugar at halftime or whenever you have time on the bench. If you play defense or goalie, keep a Gatorade behind the net just in case you need a quick burst of sugar.

Tennis: This sport is very high intensity and requires close blood sugar monitoring because you never come off the court (and also cannot rely on anyone else because you are either by yourself or with one other person, if playing doubles). There are a good number of breaks in this sport, but I would still start your blood sugar somewhere around 200, maybe even a little higher (210–225), if you are playing outside and it is really hot.

Track and Field: It is kind of difficult to speak about track and field since there are so many individual events that are really distinct from one another. However, none of the events last too long, and you should have plenty of time before and after to check your blood sugar levels. Start your blood sugar a little above 150, unless you are running long distance, in which case I advise you to start closer to 200. If you have multiple events, you can also start a little higher (175–200), and make sure you test and rest between events. If you have a long enough break between two events, try to eat a snack with some complex carbs, like a granola bar, mini sandwich, or banana.

Volleyball: I never realized what an intense sport volleyball was until I watched my high school girls' team play it. Having said that, there are a lot of time-outs, like basketball, and there is also time for you to catch your breath and regroup between sets. Start your blood sugar somewhere between 175 and 200. Volleyball is always played in a hot environment as well (either inside on a court or outside on the beach), which can cause your blood sugar levels to drop, so remain mindful of that factor.

Whether you are playing an intense soccer game or just hitting some golf balls for fun, physical activity can make it difficult to manage your T1D. Every activity and sport comes with its own set of challenges, but regardless of the obstacles, you should never let your T1D stop you from being active and having fun. If you listen to your body, keep track of your blood sugar, and plan ahead, there is no reason for T1D to be the limiting factor of your enjoyment and success in athletics.

10

TRAVELING WITH T1D

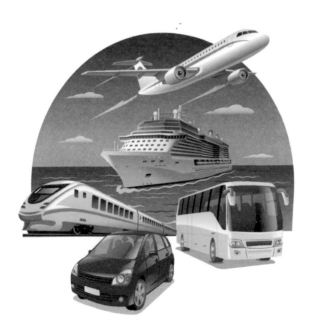

One of the few aspects of daily life that we forget to pay attention to when discussing T1D management is traveling with T1D. Whether it is driving a car or flying on a plane, traveling with T1D requires thought and care. Some forms of travel are quite simple in nature, while others require more planning. In this chapter, I will go through each mode of transportation and how you can best prepare for all of your travels, and then also provide you with some tips on how to manage your T1D while away from home.

AUTOMOBILE

Without a doubt, the most common mode of transportation is the automobile. Once you get your license, you will enter a world of freedom and adulthood. But with freedom comes responsibility. There are the regular responsibilities that come with a car: wearing a seatbelt, driving the speed limit, obeying the road signs—basic safety rules. In addition to these responsibilities, however, as a person with T1D, you have to be aware of a couple of extra safety precautions.

The first safety measure to take is making sure you have extra supplies in case an unexpected situation arises. You can never predict what is going to happen when you are on the road. I once took a five-hour trip to upstate New York, and my car broke down three hours into the trip. I was stuck on the side of the highway for thirty minutes before a tow truck finally came to rescue me. During that time, I got a low blood sugar and had no way to travel to a place to get a source of sugar. Luckily, I had a bottle of glucose tablets with me and could correct my blood sugar right then and there. Had I not been prepared for the possibility of a low blood sugar, I probably would have had to call for an ambulance. These supplies should be stored together in an easily accessible place and should be assembled before you even sit in the driver's seat. Here is a list of supplies I advise you to keep in your car at all times whenever you drive.

- *Sugar Supply*: This can be in the form of juice, candy, or glucose tablets. I prefer glucose tablets because the bottle is relatively small, but it holds enough sugar to correct more than twelve low blood sugar episodes (provided you buy a fifty-count bottle and use four glucose tablets per correction).

- *Testing Supplies*: I always keep an extra BG meter, lancets (finger prickers), and test strips in my car in case I lose the ones I normally carry with me or something breaks. Be mindful though: many BG meters will not work below 40°F, and test strips can be sensitive to extreme temperatures as well. This would be an item I suggest bringing with you when you leave your car.

- *Fast-Acting Insulin*: I would not advise keeping this in your car if it is going to be subjected to extreme temperature changes (summer heat and winter cold). However, having some fast-acting insulin like NovoLog or Humalog is a good backup in case your pump stops working or your insulin for daily injections goes bad or gets lost.

- *Emergency Glucagon Kit*: This is really important to keep in any vehicle you drive frequently. I would advise you to keep this in a location that is really close to you, like the pocket in the driver's side door or the glove compartment (somewhere a third party could easily locate if something were to happen to you). Similar to the warning I gave about testing supplies, emergency glucagon kits are not built for extreme temperatures and should not come into extended contact with direct sunlight. Carry this with you when you enter and exit your car.

- *Cell Phone*: I am including this because a cell phone is your absolute last plan in case anything goes wrong. You can always call your parents or friends if you are having troubles and are close to home, or, if matters get worse, you can call 911.

Instead of leaving these supplies in your vehicle, some people carry many, if not all, of these supplies with them already in a "go bag," which they bring with them wherever they go. If you create one of these bags, you do not need to keep all of the listed supplies in your car. Just make sure you never forget your bag when you get into your vehicle. This is a great alternative to leaving your supplies in your car because it eliminates any worry about the materials that are sensitive to temperature and sunlight (testing supplies, insulin, and emergency glucagon kit), which can go bad.

The next piece of advice I have for you is to always check your blood sugar before you start driving. It is one thing to be a passenger in a car and have the freedom to test and correct your blood sugar whenever you want. If you are driving, however, you do not have this freedom. Test your blood sugar and make any corrections you need to make before you get behind the wheel.

Having said that, there will probably come a time when you are behind the wheel and feel your blood sugar starting to rise or drop. When you feel any symptoms of either low or high blood sugars, you should pull over immediately. Driving while your blood sugar levels are irregular can impair your function, just like driving drunk. You lose focus and reaction time, which can be really dangerous to you, other people in your vehicle, and other drivers on the road. If you ignore the symptoms of low or high blood sugars or try to postpone dealing with them until you arrive at your destination, you are risking your life as well as the lives of others. Be smart and put your health and safety first.

If you are going to be driving for a long time, like the five-hour trips I make between my home in Connecticut and the college I attend in Vermont, take periodic breaks to check your blood sugar. Driving for too long without testing your blood sugar will surely lead to either a low or high blood sugar. For reference, I normally stop and test my blood sugar after every two hours of driving. It takes five minutes to pull over, park your car, and test your blood sugar; no big deal. I also use these regimented breaks to get out of the car, stretch my legs, and use the restroom, which can be quite relieving when traveling long distances.

BOATS/TRAINS/BUSES

Boats, trains, and buses are all pretty similar in that you are a passenger instead of a driver. These modes of transportation might also be common for people who live in the city or near the water. The amount of time you spend on any of these vehicles can vary, at which point you have to adjust how you manage your T1D. In the case of a short ride, make sure you have enough supplies with you for short-term use; this would include your BG meter kit, sugar source, and emergency glucagon kit. If you are taking a short ride, you do not necessarily need a whole extra supply of insulin with you. The sugar source and emergency glucagon kit are extremely important, though. Just like transportation in an automobile, life can be very unpredictable, so you need to be prepared for anything and everything.

Longer rides on any of these modes of transportation require a bit more attention. For a long bus, train, or ferry ride, make sure you have the items I just listed, plus extra insulin and/or pump sites you will need for the duration of your trip. During my freshman year of high school, I went on a bus trip with my school band to Universal Studios in Florida and packed a whole extra bag for my T1D materials. Along the same lines, make sure that your supplies always stay close to you during your travels. Do not put extra supplies in the carry space below a bus when you are going on a long trip; you will not have access to them if you should need them. This happened to me on our bus trip down to Florida, and I was lucky to have a friend with T1D who was also on the trip and who let me use some of her supplies. If you have to, tell the driver to stop whatever mode of transportation you are on so you can access your supplies. Of course, it would probably be much simpler to just keep your supplies with you and avoid that kind of situation entirely. If you are on a boat and there is a chance that the weather will be pretty hot, make sure any insulin you bring with you is stored in a place where it will not overheat.

AIRPLANES

A few additional steps are required for people with T1D when traveling on airplanes. First, double-check to make sure all of your

T1D supplies are in your carry-on luggage and not the luggage you plan on checking in that will go in the cargo hold of the plane. Just like anywhere else, you always want to have access to your T1D supplies in case you need them. In addition, recall that there is a long duration of time when you will be completely separated from the luggage you check in. You can never be 100 percent positive what will happen from the time you drop it off to the time you pick it up. If anything were to get "lost" from your luggage on your flight from, say, New York City to Mexico, it would be very difficult to find replacement medicine without having to jump through a multitude of hoops, especially in a foreign country. Luggage does actually get lost sometimes, and the last thing you want is to be looking for your luggage that contains all your T1D supplies after you land, only to find out it actually never made it onto the plane.

The next thing you need to be aware of is security. Security has gotten very strict recently, and as a result, people with T1D have to do a bit more work in order to convince security that we need all of the medical supplies in our bags. To stay in compliance and make everything as easy as possible, try to pack all of your T1D supplies in clear, plastic bags. Most of the time, security will see the needles and insulin in your bag and not even ask you about it. They are trained to see these items and usually know what looks normal and what does not. Still, I play it on the safe side and always say to the security individual nearest me, "Hello. I just wanted to let you know that I have type 1 diabetes, and I have needles and insulin in my bag. Is there anyone else I need to inform about this?" Even with these precautions, if you are still nervous about getting through security at an airport, you can always have your diabetes doctor send you a note that you can print out and bring with you on the trip: "Patrick McAllister has type 1 diabetes and needs his insulin, BG meter, emergency glucagon kit, and sugar source to properly take care of his blood sugar levels. Carrying these items on his person at all times is essential to his health and well-being. —Dr. John Smith."

From my traveling experience, security officials seem to have less trouble with my insulin and needles and more trouble with the liquids I am carrying (e.g., juice boxes). I went through a security checkpoint in JFK International Airport on my way to see a Notre Dame football game with my friends and our fathers, and security officials stopped me because I was carrying juice boxes in my bag. Apparently, the juice boxes contained more than the maximum 3.4 oz. of fluids allowed on an airplane, so they had to run a test on each individual juice box to make sure I was not trying to transport anything illegal. It was a hassle, but I understand why they had to take precautions. To prevent this, I suggest traveling with glucose tablets; they are really compact and will not prompt airport security to stop you for questioning.

MANAGING YOUR T1D IN UNFAMILIAR PLACES

While this chapter is mainly supposed to help you manage your T1D while traveling, I feel compelled to talk a little about how to manage your T1D once you've gotten to your destination. Obviously, this section does not apply to those thirty-minute car rides to your grandmother's house or twenty-minute trips by bus with your soccer team to a rival school, but if you happen to be traveling to somewhere unknown, such as a different state or country, there are certain precautions you should take to ensure your T1D does not stop you from having a good time.

The first piece of advice for long-distance travel to a largely unfamiliar place is to pack double the amount of supplies you think you will need. You can never predict what might happen on an extended trip and how difficult it might be to replace your supplies should you happen to lose them. Many foreign countries do not have access to the same medical supplies we do, which can make getting even something as common as insulin rather difficult. Along with planning ahead by packing extra T1D supplies, you might want to also think about packing extra snacks if you are entering a new culture, especially if you are unaccustomed to how many carbs are in their foods and drinks.

Another smart idea is to make an appointment with your diabetes doctor prior to leaving for your trip. Inform your doctors that you will be in a different location for an extended amount of time so they can help you plan how to best manage your T1D. Some important topics to discuss with them are:

- Changes in injection or pump regimens because of a change in time zone
- Increasing blood sugar testing frequency in a new place with a new routine
- Additional immunizations that might be recommended for the place you are traveling to
- A well-thought-out "sick-day" plan in case of traveler's diarrhea or stomach bug
- A list of contact information comprised of your doctors, nutritionists, and anyone else you might need to contact in case you need help managing your T1D while traveling.

No matter what mode of transportation you are taking or where in the world you are traveling to, staying alert is key. You have to pay close attention to your blood sugar because you are no longer in the comfort of your own home with your usual resources available to you. If you are traveling with others, make sure you let them know you have T1D and what to do in case of an emergency (show them your emergency glucagon kit). If you are traveling alone, I would only tell someone if you are traveling long distance, such as a long bus ride or a plane ride. Inform the bus driver or one of the flight attendants just so someone around you knows you have T1D, should anything happen. Additionally, this is where wearing a medical bracelet or necklace with your information on it is extremely important. If you stick to your regimen and the guidelines I just outlined, your T1D should not hinder your ability to travel in the slightest.

11

SEX, DRUGS, AND ROCK 'N' ROLL

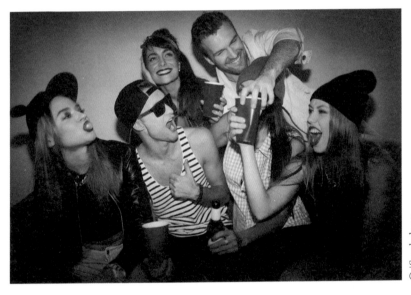

As you can probably tell from the title, this chapter will cover some of the most underdiscussed topics involving T1D. Having conversations about these topics with your parents and diabetes providers can be especially difficult. Your parents love you and always want you to be safe, and several of these topics outwardly defy that. Similarly, you may not know your doctors well enough to feel comfortable asking them questions regarding these topics. I guess this is where my book may come in especially handy. Regardless of how uneasy or awkward some of these topics can be, they are all extremely important to discuss if you want to be able to manage your T1D in the real world.

SEX

I figured a good place to start would be with one of the most awkward topics; after this point, nothing will seem as uncomfortable. Before we begin, if you are planning on reading this section and have no idea what sex even is, I would highly suggest reading a book about sex and health prior to continuing. Knowing a bit of information before reading my tips on how to manage sex with T1D will make understanding the material much easier.

Another point I would like to make is that I am not giving you tips for how to manage sex with T1D because I believe that sex is a requirement of life. I completely understand that some of you might not be sexually active yet while others have no intention of becoming sexually active. That is okay. Choosing to be sexually active or not is just that: a choice. If you are not currently sexually active, some of this information might not be relevant to you, and there is no shame in that. My intentions for discussing this topic are to give you tips and advice in case the time comes when you decide to become sexually active.

Sex is a passionate and intimate activity you commonly share with someone you really care about. Sometimes you get so "into it" that you feel like nothing else in the world matters. Unfortunately, this mindset can be a major downfall for people with T1D. Because you have T1D, you always have to remain aware of what your body is telling you. You never know when something might happen that will cause your blood sugar to spike or drop, even during sex. If you are about to have sex with someone, you should check your blood sugar beforehand. I know how ridiculous this sounds, but trust me, you would much rather correct a low blood sugar before you are "physically invested" as opposed to during the act.

Having said that, I understand that it is not always possible (or realistic) to test your blood sugar before having sex. On top of being passionate and intimate, sex is also often spontaneous. This is one of the many reasons why people with T1D should always carry a sugar source with them in case a situation arises that might cause them to have a low blood sugar.

Another fundamental fact about sex is that it is a physical activity. Sex generally requires a sizable amount of energy, depending on how long and how intensely you are having sex. Just like every other physical activity, sex can cause your blood sugar to drop. If you happen to be in the middle of having sex and you feel your blood sugar going low, you must stop immediately and correct. I know how hard it can be (believe me), but it is something you *have* to do. From my experience, once the crappy low blood sugar feelings start taking over, sex is no longer enjoyable anyway. Additionally, as I have said many times before, make sure you let enough time pass before "starting up" again. I know all you are probably thinking about when you are waiting for your blood sugar to rise is getting back to having sex, but you need to let your body recover. If you give your body the proper amount of time, you will have no problem whatsoever getting back "into the groove."

One of the common questions some of my close friends ask me about sex and T1D is, "How does your girlfriend handle the whole thing?" First, if you are having sex with someone, you should undoubtedly tell him or her that you have T1D. I will assume you will be alone with your partner when having sex, which therefore makes your partner the only person who can help you if something goes wrong with your blood sugar. Give your partner a brief overview of what T1D is and what he or she can do in certain situations. Do not be nervous about telling your partner you have T1D. If you are at the point in a relationship where you are having sex with someone, you should certainly feel comfortable enough to tell him or her (for tips on how and what to tell someone you have T1D, refer to chapter 7, "Telling People You Know").

If you are in the middle of having sex and feel your blood sugar dropping, it is perfectly okay to tell your partner that you need to take a break and test your blood sugar. He or she will understand and will probably even offer to help. My girlfriend in high school and college was great about this. Whenever we had sex and I had to stop because of a low blood sugar, she always asked me where my juice boxes or glucose tablets were so she could get them for me. I never had to ask her for help, and I don't think she felt burdened or obligated to help me either. In fact, most of the time I was able to correct my blood sugar without her assistance, but that does not change how refreshing it was to see how much she cared about me. I am sure your partner will react in the same way that my girlfriend did for me.

Sex can be a tricky activity to manage with your T1D. You must always remain mindful of your how you are feeling before, during, and after having sex. If you can do this and follow the guidelines I set out in this section, your T1D should not hinder you in the slightest from having sex.

DRUGS

Drug use, like sex, is a rather taboo topic to discuss with respect to T1D management. To preface this section, I want to start by making it perfectly clear that I will only be discussing a couple drugs in this section, namely marijuana and alcohol. These two drugs are prominent in our society and very hard to avoid. On top of that, both of these drugs are on the weaker end of the "drug spectrum." What you will *not* find in this section is my advice on how to handle harder drugs, such as cocaine, heroin, LSD, ecstasy, or crystal meth. If you are considering trying any of these drugs, T1D is the least of your problems. Besides the fact that they are all illegal, these drugs are addictive and can *kill you*. If that does not stop you from wanting to try these drugs, then I do not know what will.

Similar to our discussion on sex, I would also like to note that I am not writing this section with the suggestion that smoking marijuana and drinking alcohol are requirements of teenage life. Up to this point, I am twenty-two years old and have never smoked marijuana or gotten so blackout drunk that I lost control of my body and mind. My rationale for abstaining from avid marijuana and alcohol use is that I have an easier time controlling my blood sugar and overall health than I would if those two factors were a greater part of my life. Having said this, the information in this next section on how to manage your T1D while using drugs comes largely from my conversations with my friends who have T1D who have had ample experience with marijuana and alcohol. Their experiences, combined with my knowledge of the human body and information I have been given by doctors and nutritionists, allows me to have complete confidence in the advice I am about to give you.

Let's talk a little about what marijuana and alcohol have in common and how they affect your T1D. From my experience and basic knowledge about how drugs work, people take drugs for one main reason—to feel better than they already feel. Drugs alter your state of mind to a point where you are no longer totally in control of your mind and body. Some people really like being in this altered state of mind. However, this can be dangerous for people with T1D. Not having complete control of your mind means you are not conscious about how your body feels (i.e., low or high blood sugars). If you decide to use drugs, my first piece of advice is to be smart, plain and simple. Set alarms to remind yourself to check your blood sugar and take insulin. Tell a sober friend that you are going to drink or get high so he or she can keep an eye on you. Plan these things out ahead of time while you are still sober so that if you decide to get high or drunk, you will not have to worry about it when you are in an altered state of mind.

MARIJUANA (WEED)

Marijuana use has increased significantly in the past years because of changing legislation, decriminalization, and even legalization, making it readily available almost anywhere you go. If you decide to use marijuana and get high, there are a few specifics you have to be careful of.

As I mentioned in the introduction to this section, one of the main concerns with drugs and T1D is the fact that drugs can alter your state of mind and therefore make you forgetful about your T1D-related responsibilities. Weed *definitely* alters your state of mind. The main drug in weed responsible for its psychological effects on you is **THC (tetrahydrocannabinol)**. It gets into your brain and does all kinds of weird stuff, making you feel funky. To combat the effects of the THC, set alarms to test your blood sugar and take insulin. You should also inform a friend that you are going to get high, which will probably not be a problem since you will most likely be getting high in the company of other people. Have your friend set alarms too. In addition, make sure your T1D supplies are near you, as you will probably have trouble finding them (or having the motivation to find them) when you are high. Create these backup plans before you get high so you do not have to worry about it once the high starts to kick in.

Weed can be smoked, vaporized, and eaten, all of which do the same thing to your body, but with different intensities. In terms of carb counting, the only form of weed that needs to be taken into consideration is edibles, the form that is eaten. Usually, people will consume weed in the form of brownies or gummies, both of which have tons of carbs. Make sure you account for those carbs if you decide to consume them.

The last thing I will say when it comes to dealing with weed and T1D is to be extra careful when counting carbs when you are high. An all-too-common term associated with weed is "the munchies," referring to the fact that weed can make you exceptionally hungry. Many people, including people with T1D, lose track of what exactly they eat when they are high. Try especially hard not to let this happen to you. Unlike everyone else, you need to take insulin based on how many carbs you eat. This is another instance where setting alarms can be extremely helpful—they will hopefully snap you back into reality for a couple seconds to realize you have to take your insulin. Having said this, make sure you do not over-bolus and take too much insulin to counteract carbs that you might not have. Trying to correct a low blood sugar while high can prove much more difficult than in normal situations, so avoiding that scenario altogether is definitely preferable. One of my friends who has T1D and who smokes weed fairly often has told me that counting carbs and taking the correct amount of insulin for those carbs is by far the hardest part of T1D management when high. Fortunately for him, he has also told me that he can still feel both high and low blood sugars when high, so he is able to respond accordingly if his blood sugar levels drop or spike. Knowing this, however, do not assume that you will automatically be able to feel your blood sugar levels change when high. Some people can stay in touch with their senses better than others. If you decide to get high, you need to plan as if you will not be able to feel your blood sugar spike or drop, so that you are ready for any and every possibility.

ALCOHOL

Just as weed comes with its fair share of challenges when trying to manage your T1D, so does alcohol. Alcohol can affect your body and how it uses insulin and processes carbs, as well as your ability to recognize and correct irregular blood sugar levels. On top of that, there are thousands of different alcoholic drinks out there, all of which are mixed with different ingredients (many of them super sugary), which can also have a dangerous impact on your blood sugar levels.

One of my friends who has T1D once threw a party in his dorm room during college. He drank a bunch of alcohol that night and passed out on the floor of his dorm room. His roommate came in about twenty minutes later and, remembering that he had T1D, called 911. When the ambulance got to his room, his blood sugar was 43. He had a hypoglycemic event (low blood sugar) that caused him to pass out because the alcohol had made him incapable of feeling his symptoms and treating his blood sugar. On top of that, other people at the party just walked right by him because they assumed he had passed out because he was drunk. Luckily for him, he had informed his roommate about his T1D before the party, which ended up saving his life. This story is not meant to scare you but rather to show you how fine the line is between life and death if you have T1D and drink. I am not saying don't drink; I am just saying that if you decide to drink, be careful.

The best piece of advice to help prevent a scary scenario like this is to check your blood sugar frequently. I know it can be a pain, and even more so when you are drinking and trying to have a good time, but it is your responsibility to take care of yourself. Set alarms, tell friends to remind you, or use some other method to keep your blood sugar on the right path. It is much easier to play the "prevention" game than the "oh, crap, I feel really low" game.

Another commonality with all types of alcohol is how the alcohol itself can affect the insulin in your body. Alcohol intake can lead to lower blood sugar levels because it impacts the liver's ability to release glucose into your bloodstream. What this means is that if your blood sugar were to start going low, your body may not respond appropriately. Couple this with the fact that you won't be able to sense low blood sugar levels in the same way because of the alcohol's effect on your brain, and you are at risk for a really intense low blood sugar reaction.

For this reason, doctors frequently advise patients not to account for any carbs in the alcohol when deciding how much insulin to bolus. However, you still have to pay attention to how much food you eat when you drink, as well as certain mixers that may be filled with sugar. I will discuss how to deal with different types of alcohols and mixtures later in this chapter.

One of the more hectic situations you might have to deal with when drinking, and more specifically if you are drunk, is vomiting. Vomiting is no fun for anyone, but it can be especially dangerous for people with T1D. If you drink enough alcohol and start vomiting, all of the "stuff" you are puking into the toilet (or onto the floor of someone's basement) might not be solely alcohol. Your vomit could contain food from earlier in the day—food your body was going to digest but did not have the chance to. Vomiting can cause blood sugar levels to drop significantly because it leaves your body with a lack of carbs and an excess of insulin. If you are vomiting and do not feel that you have the means to get your blood sugar under control, I would definitely suggest calling an ambulance and taking a trip to the emergency room. This is *not* something you want to play around with. Vomiting can cause serious problems for people with T1D, so do not take the situation lightly if it arises.

In this next section, I will go over how to deal with counting carbs of specific alcohols and mixtures, as well as a few types of alcohol you should try to avoid.

ALCOHOL (AND COMPANY) AND ITS IMPACT ON YOUR BLOOD SUGAR

As you may know, there are many different types of alcohol: beer, vodka, rum, and wine—just to name a few. Each of these can affect your blood sugar differently, usually dependent on what else you are drinking with that alcohol. Let's go through the list:

Beer: Even though beer is made from grain, which contains carbs, you should *not* count any of the carbs in beer when deciding how much insulin to give yourself.

Wine: Wine is similar to beer in the sense that even though it may taste sugary or sweet in some cases, you should not account for any of the carbs in the wine you are drinking when calculating for a bolus.

Hard Liquor (Vodka/Rum/Tequila/Whiskey): These types of alcohol are similar to beer and wine in the sense that you should refrain from counting the carbs in the liquor when totaling the number of carbs to bolus for. However, the catch with hard alcohol is that when it is taken via a shot, it is often paired with a "chaser," which commonly contains carbs that you will have to account for (see "chasers" section below).

Mixed Drinks: These drinks are usually a mix of a hard alcohol and something sweet, such as juice or soda. Common mixed drinks include but are by no means limited to margaritas, mojitos, mimosas, piña coladas, daiquiris, and fruity martinis. Unless you know how many carbs are in the drink that is being mixed with the alcohol you are drinking, avoid drinking it. Mixed drinks are common at bars and clubs and are also made slightly differently every time. Even if the bartender seems confident, I doubt he or she knows exactly how many carbs are in the drink they just made (I am a bartender, and the majority of the time I have no idea). Another common example of a dangerous mixed drink is the infamous "jungle juice" at college parties. There is absolutely no way of figuring out what is in that big punch bowl in the corner of the room, so save yourself the trouble and stick with drinks you either brought to the party yourself or that were given to you with the cap still on.

CHASERS

Chasers are drinks that you pair with hard alcohols. The idea behind a chaser is that because hard alcohol is so "hard" to swallow, you need something less severe to wash it down with. Sometimes beer is used as a chaser, but more commonly chasers are really sugary drinks, such as soda or juice. As we know from our earlier discussion on carbs, juice and soda contain *lots* of carbs and tend to spike your blood sugar, especially because they are liquids and will enter your system quickly.

If you plan on drinking hard alcohol with a sugary chaser, you have to be extremely careful that you count the carbs in the chaser. Additionally, you need to be very thoughtful about how much insulin you are going to take for a chaser, as the juice/soda often impacts your blood glucose faster than the insulin can work. This is a set up for a low blood sugar reaction.

As an individual with T1D, you should try to avoid chasers because it is just too difficult to keep track of all the carbs in the chaser combined with how the alcohol is going to affect your blood sugar. In addition, it can be quite difficult limiting yourself to only drinking your chaser after a shot of liquor. I have seen people run out of their chasers countless times because they were passively drinking more of the chaser than they were their actual alcoholic beverage.

ROCK 'N' ROLL (PARTIES)

It only makes sense to follow up a section about managing your T1D with alcohol with one that discusses how to manage your T1D at parties. The word *party* is pretty ambiguous and covers a wide range of gatherings—everything from your little cousin's birthday party to the midnight rager in your friend's basement. For the purposes of this chapter, I will be discussing more of the "rager in your friend's basement" kind of parties.

One of the first things that you should check off your list when at a party is to make sure that at least one other person present knows you have T1D. Your parents or guardians will probably not be in attendance, so you will need to make sure a trusted friend is aware of your T1D. This is just a precautionary detail I always include, but it can really save you in the long run. If you look back in the alcohol section, you will recall my friend whose life was saved because someone else at his college dorm party knew he had T1D and was able to get him help before it was too late.

Keeping along the lines of planning and preventing, my next piece of advice is to make sure your T1D supplies are on your person at all times. I once went to a party in high school and left my T1D supplies in my backpack, which I had dropped off at the front door of the house. Some thirty minutes later, I felt a low blood sugar coming on, and I left my friends to get my BG meter out of my backpack only to find that my backpack was not where I had left it. I spent the next ten minutes freaking out, unable to find my supplies, until the kid who lived at the house finally told me he had moved my backpack into a closet so people would not trip on it. It was a scary feeling, and ever since then, I make sure I know exactly where my T1D supplies are when I am at a party.

The Big Two: Food and Alcohol

There are always two common themes at basically all parties of this nature: food and alcohol. Let us start with food. It is *so* easy to forget about counting carbs when at a party; I have done this more times than I can remember. The big bowl of tortilla chips and salsa is just sitting on the table in the middle of the room, and it is common practice to take a handful every time you walk by (which I seem to do about every thirty seconds). This will be hard, but I urge you, save yourself the trouble and find some way to remind yourself to test your blood sugar and correct for all the carbs you are eating. No one is saying that you have to completely avoid party snack food because you have T1D; just make sure you account for it. Additionally, there are options on many insulin pumps to program an extended bolus that allows for grazing over a set time period. You might want to talk to your diabetes provider to see if this bolus option will work for you.

Now, for the alcohol. I talked extensively about how alcohol can affect your T1D earlier in this chapter, but I would like to reiterate something I briefly touched on: *jungle juice*—the massive bowl in the center of parties, consisting of a mixture of hard liquors and really sugary drinks (fruit punch, Gatorade, Kool-Aid, etc.). Jungle juice is a really bad idea for people with T1D (and all people in general). It is named *jungle juice* because when people drink it, they turn into animals. Even the people that make the jungle juice do not know exactly what is in it, which is an immediate red flag for me. If you do not know how much sugar is in something, it is going to be pretty difficult to take the correct amount of insulin for it. Steer clear of the jungle juice and stick to the drinks that you actually know the contents of.

Dancing with T1D

One of the last things I will say in reference to parties is a factor people commonly overlook: dancing. I love dancing! It is a great way to let loose and have fun with your friends. Having said that, there are several ways dancing can really affect your blood sugar. For one, dancing is a physical activity, which, as you know by now, means you are consuming sugar at a faster rate in order to give yourself the energy to successfully perform the dougie or electric slide.

On top of your body using up energy to execute all of your impressive dance moves, your body also has to expend energy to thermoregulate. When you are dancing, you are probably squeezed into a small area with a bunch of other hot and sweaty people. Your body has to use energy to maintain the right temperature in comparison to the outside world. This can lead to lower blood sugar levels, so beware. I came to this realization at prom during my senior year of high school. I was on the dance floor "busting a move," when I suddenly got that weird stomachache feeling that screams, "*Low blood sugar!*" I stopped dancing, sat down to test my blood sugar, and found that I was 45. *How did this happen?* I had not taken any insulin yet because I had not eaten anything; all I had were a few glasses of Diet Coke. After taking a couple of glucose tablets and resting for ten minutes, I realized that it was the dancing that had caused my blood sugar to drop. Take it from me, if you are going to dance at a party, check your blood sugar before you head out onto the dance floor. Get some sugar into your system if you have to, and then get out there and represent the T1D Nation with your stellar dance moves.

12

OFF TO COLLEGE WITH T1D

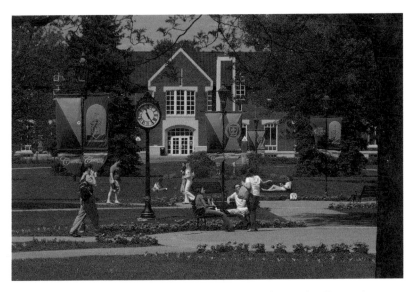

Saint Michael's College. Used with permission from Alex Bertoni.

Up to this point, we have discussed the ins and outs of managing T1D during childhood and adolescence. Do not mistake any of the information in the previous chapters as trivial; counting carbs, dealing with sick days, and managing your blood sugar while playing sports are all difficult situations to be able to control. However, keep in mind that for the most part, all of these situations have occurred with your home and family nearby. Even as a person who manages his T1D fairly independently, I realize that being close to my house and parents makes everything a lot easier. Being able to come home and know when you are having dinner and exactly how many carbs are in that dinner is a luxury. Much of this changes when you go off to college.

Now, do not let this initial statement discourage you from going away to college. College can be one of the greatest experiences of your life. It is a time when you are given more freedom than you have ever been given before. You will finally start learning what interests you in school, and you will have the freedom to meet new people and explore new places. Having said this, for many people, myself included, college is the first time you spend an extended period of time away from home and away from your family. This can be scary. Not having your parents to lean on or your friends to hang out with can be pretty overwhelming. And we have not even added T1D into the equation yet.

The transition to college can be a difficult one, but my goal in this chapter is to make your struggles of going off to college *not* T1D related. I remember my first year at college very vividly and will lay out everything you need to know in order to make your transition to college with T1D simple and straightforward.

MOVING OUT

The first logical thing you will have to do is move out of your own house and into a college dorm. In the next two sections, I will give you tips on things to keep in mind when you are moving out of your house and into your new room. First, if you are planning to go to a college that is far away from your home, do not stress. The distance between your house and college should play only a minuscule role in your ability to manage your T1D. I go to Saint Michael's College (which is about five hours away from my family's house), and I have never had a T1D-related problem that could have been avoided if I were closer to home. The only real effect that distance has in your

T1D life is your accessibility to your diabetes doctor (endocrinologist) in person. I will go over how to manage being far away from your endocrinologist a little later in this chapter.

When moving out of your house, there are a few essential items you need to remember to bring with you. Most of them will probably seem obvious, but feel free to use this list as a checklist when moving out:

- *Insulin*: Do not let it get too cold or too hot during your moving process. Store it in a mini cooler when traveling to prevent its exposure to extreme temperatures.
- *BG Meters*: Bring multiple so you have backups.
- *Pump Materials*: infusion sites, pump, and extra batteries
- *Alcohol Wipes*: for daily insulin injections or pump injections
- *Emergency Glucose Supplies*: inclusive of glucagon kits and glucose gels
- *Minifridge*: If you do not already have one of these, you should buy one for college. Most freshman dorm rooms do not come with a fridge, and you need a place to store your insulin.
- *Sugar Supplies*: inclusive of glucose tablets, juice boxes, and other stuff to correct your low blood sugars
- *Prescription Information*: so you can order prescriptions at college (I will talk about how to do this later in the chapter)
- *Insurance Card*: also for ordering prescriptions

Another tip is to make sure all of your T1D supplies are easily accessible during the entire trip to college. When I was moving out to go to Saint Mike's, I accidently packed my T1D supplies first when squeezing everything into our family van. We were halfway up to Saint Mike's from Connecticut and stopped for breakfast at some local diner in southern Vermont. When I pulled out my insulin pen from my backpack to give myself an injection, I realized it was empty. I opened up the back of our van to get a replacement pen, but had to rummage past all of my clothes, shoes, and school materials that were also jammed into the back of the van. When all was said and done, it took about thirty minutes to pull everything out of the van, locate my T1D supplies, and then load everything back in. Luckily, I was not in a rush to get the supplies. This would have been a completely different story if I needed to get some emergency glucose gel because I was experiencing a dangerously low blood sugar. The moral of the story is to pack your T1D supplies in a place where you can easily access them.

The last thing I will say about moving out to college is to create a T1D contact list. This list should be composed of anyone who might not be in your saved contact list on your phone but who you might need to contact while at college with T1D-related questions or concerns. Names and telephone numbers I have put in my list include the following:

- primary care doctor's office
- diabetes doctor's office
- nutritionist
- pharmacy (both at home and one close to my college)
- any relatives or family friends who live near my college (in case I need immediate help from someone I trust while at college)

At some point during your time at college, you may need these names and phone numbers. It is always better to have these contacts organized and available than to have to search all over the place when you actually need them. Keep the contact list in your phone as well as in a desk drawer or some other accessible place in your dorm room.

MOVING IN/ESTABLISHING YOURSELF ON CAMPUS

For the most part, moving out is pretty straightforward. You just have to remember to pack everything you need, and possibly purchase a couple supplies along the way (like extra juice boxes and a minifridge). Moving into college, however, can be a little bit trickier. You are in a new environment, and there is an assortment of housekeeping things you have to take care of. I will explain in detail each of the steps you should take when moving in.

First, actually move in. Get everything unloaded from your cars and place them in your dorm room. Unpack your minifridge and get it pumping. Since your dorm room will probably be pretty hot and sticky (unless you have air conditioning, in which case I envy you), your insulin will be susceptible to degradation. Even way up north in Vermont at Saint Michael's College, it must have been 90°F when I moved into my dorm room. After loosely unpacking, I left my room without setting up my minifridge and accidently left some of my insulin pens on my desk for a couple hours in the heat. When I returned later in the day, they were steaming hot and I had to throw them out. A good idea might be to crank up the temperature all of the way on your mini-fridge when you first move in to get it cold fast—just don't do this with your insulin inside because it could freeze if the temperature drops too quickly. After unpacking, the next things on your to-do list can be done in any order, but within the first couple days of moving in.

Roommate

First on this list is meeting your roommate and telling him or her about your T1D. If you are having trouble with the nuances of informing your roommate about your T1D, see chapter 7, "Telling People You Know." When informing your roommate, make sure you teach him or her how to use the emergency glucagon kit. There will be many times when your roommate will be the only one around you, so he or she definitely needs to be equipped to handle an emergency situation, should one arise. It might seem a bit overwhelming to inform your roommate about all of this serious T1D stuff before he or she even gets to know your favorite TV show, but trust me, if you are passed out on the ground, the fact that your roommate knows you love *Game of Thrones* will not help you one bit.

I also understand if you are concerned that informing your roommate that you have T1D might affect your relationship. In a completely new environment surrounded by nothing but strangers, the last thing you want to do is scare off the first person you meet, who also happens to be the person you are going to be living with for the upcoming year. When I moved in, I was definitely nervous about telling my freshman roommate, Mike, about my T1D. Looking back though, it could not have gone any better. He was completely understanding and asked me probably fifty times within the first week if there was anything he could to do help me. He knew a couple of people from his hometown who had T1D and was familiar with how they managed it. Needless to say, Mike remained my roommate throughout my remaining four years at Saint Mike's. I am hopeful that your roommate will be just as understanding and helpful to you as Mike was to me.

In the less ideal scenario where you find yourself in an unfortunate situation and your roommate is insensitive to your T1D, there is nothing wrong with going to your residence life office on campus and requesting a room switch. Your safety and comfort should come above all else, and if your roommate makes you feel unsafe or uncomfortable, you have every right to get out of that room and into one with a roommate who is more accommodating.

One thing that really helped me establish a good relationship with Mike was contacting him before school actually started. Even if you opt into the random housing selection during the summer, colleges are pretty good about letting you know who your roommate is before school begins. When you get your roommate's name, go on Facebook or any other social media site and try to make contact. I talked a lot with Mike over Facebook before we met at Saint Mike's, but in all our conversations I never mentioned I had T1D. I wanted to wait until we met in person to inform him, but, looking back, it would have been better to inform him as soon as possible. If you have the opportunity, tell your roommate about your T1D before you both get on campus. This little heads-up will help prevent any awkward or surprising conversations that might take place when you meet face to face for the first time.

RA and RD

Seek out your RA (residence assistant) and RD (residence director) and also inform them about your T1D. An RA is an upperclassman who agrees to live with underclassmen and basically serves as their supervisor. The RD is usually a graduate student who agrees to the same terms, but on a larger scale. The RA is commonly attached to one hall in the residence building, while the RD is responsible for the entire building. Do not assume that your RA and RD will automatically receive information notifying them that you have T1D. On the contrary, many university stipulations prevent the health services department on campus from releasing your medical information to anyone. Knowing this, it is up to you to make contact with both your RA and RD. Telling them that you have T1D will mentally prepare them if you need help with managing your blood sugar at any time. On a side note, your RA and RD are also the "law enforcers" of your residence building, so showing them that you are a responsible and mature person might help you in case you ever get into some kind of trouble (a noise complaint, for example).

Health Services

The next thing on your agenda should be to introduce yourself to your campus's health services office. Every college has one, and this department can help you in many ways. The best course of action is to contact this office before you get on campus. Just like informing your roommate, giving your health services office a heads-up as soon as possible is always preferred. They will have your medical information regardless, so you do not have to inform them if you do not wish; however, I am sure they would appreciate it if you came in so they can match your face with the name on their list. You do not have to make a big appointment to stop in to see them, either. When I arrived on my campus, I simply walked into the office and introduced myself to a few of the nurse practitioners on staff. The conversation took no more than five minutes, and it helped me to establish a relationship with them for future visits, both T1D related and not.

Your health services office should also have empty sharps containers that you can take back to your dorm for your used lancets, needles, and old pump sites. Back home, I used to throw needles into old milk and juice cartons, but this method is much better. One container usually lasts me an entire academic year, so at the beginning of every academic year I make my stop into the health services office, say hello, and pick up my sharps container.

Accessibility Services

The next office to visit would be your school's accessibility services office. This is the office on campus that helps students with learning disabilities and accommodations. You should make someone in this office aware of your pre-existing 504 Plan, so they can help you in the rare case that one of your professors gives you a hard time. College does not abide by the same 504 Plans as middle school and high school, so, once again, it is up to you to make contact and advocate for yourself. Ideally, you should visit this office before you actually move in because it gets very busy once school starts. Most schools have the paperwork you will need on their website, so you can fill it out and send it off ahead of time with a letter from your diabetes doctor attesting to your T1D. Once your campus's accessibility services has your name on file, it is basically the same thing as having a 504 Plan—but you have to make first contact. I had the most wonderful experience when I went to my accessibility services office at Saint Mike's. One of the staff members in the office helped me with everything I needed to feel comfortable and secure on campus. The people in accessibility services offices are usually extremely friendly, and I am hopeful that the one at your college will treat you just as they treated me.

Food/Dining Services

The last department you should visit before classes start is food/dining services. This is the department that takes care of all the dining on campus. Find out where their office is and who you should meet with. With some of the other offices, you can just walk in and talk to someone, but dining services is usually pretty busy, and you will most likely have to contact someone to arrange an appointment. When you sit down to meet, first let them know who you are and that you have T1D. I am sure they will be able to inform you of all the built-in accommodations there are for people with T1D. When I sat down and talked with the director of food services my freshman year, I asked him how I would know how many carbs are in the foods they prepare. He assured me that standing cards with nutritional facts would be placed right next to each food served. Sometimes they are also available online.

The next question you might want to ask applies to the number of dining hall swipes you receive, for those of you who have this meal plan system. Luckily, I was on an unlimited meal plan my freshman year and did not have to worry about this problem, but you might need to address it if you have limited swipes. For example, there might come a time during your college career when your blood sugar drops and you have no sugar source with you; all you have is the closest dining hall. Ask the food services representative how they can help you if you need something to correct a low blood sugar, such as a juice or soda that is in the dining hall, but do not want to use one of your swipes because you are not intending to eat a full meal. I am sure they will be able to accommodate you.

A final detail: During my freshman year, food services did not allow students to bring their backpacks into the dining hall. I had a problem with this because I was still on daily injections at the time. My backpack contained all of my testing supplies and insulin, and I needed to keep them with me. I told the director of food services, and he said, "Absolutely no problem. We will introduce you to the ladies who check everyone into the dining hall, and let them know you can bring your backpack in."

The food services department, as well as every other department at Saint Mike's, was extremely nice and accommodating to me when I got onto campus. Being proactive about my health showed many of these campus services what kind of a person I was, which made them much more willing to help me. I also made it easy for them because I was friendly and responsible about every individual situation. If you go into your meetings with each campus service with a level and mature head, there is no reason why they should not accommodate your requests.

CLASSES

Once school starts, you will spend many hours in the classroom. Class subject and size can vary greatly—lecture classes at larger universities can have upwards of three hundred students in a single room, while seminar-oriented classes can have anywhere between fifteen and twenty students. My roommate Mike once had a physics class that consisted of him and only one other student! No matter what kind of classes you are enrolled in or how many students there are in your class, you have to be able to navigate through those classes with T1D. You can ensure T1D does not get in your way by making it known that you have it. Now, I am not saying to get up on top of a desk the first day of classes and make an announcement to everyone (although that would be pretty effective), but there are definitely certain people you should inform. Let's start with the most obvious: your professors.

Your professors should be among the first people you tell you have T1D once classes start, similar to how you informed your teachers in middle school and high school. If anything were to happen to you during class that would require help from someone, your professors will be the first ones to step in. That being said, if one of these situations arises, your teachers will be of little help if they do not know what is going on.

The other reason it can be important to tell your professors is so you can form a friendly relationship with each professor you have. This is another one of the few times when T1D actually gives you an advantage over everyone else. Speaking to your professors about your T1D is a great excuse to request an individual meeting with each professor and formally introduce yourself and establish a relationship. At some of the larger universities, such as the ones with the three-hundred-student lectures, it is easy to get lost in the crowd. By meeting with your professor and talking about your T1D, you will be able to showcase that you are a responsible and independent student. By just having a conversation with your professors, you will implant yourself in their minds as one of the "good" students.

At this moment, I am a senior in college, and I have met with every professor I have ever had in my college career within the first week of school. The encounter usually consists of me saying something along these lines:

> "I have had T1D since I was twelve, and I have a pretty good handle on it. If you see me testing my blood sugar or leaving your class for a couple of minutes, I am probably just correcting an irregular blood sugar. I figured I would just let you know so that we are on the same page."

In addition to telling your professors you have T1D, it is usually a good idea to tell at least one other student in your classes as well, preferably someone who sits near you. You will probably make friends in each of your classes, and in many cases, those people will be in multiple classes with you since you both will probably have the same major. A core group of four to five students who are in all of my classes know I have T1D. It just makes me feel more comfortable and safe to know that there are other people aware of my T1D, should I need help.

FINDING A LOCAL DOCTOR

One of the topics my parents and I spoke about at length when we knew I would be going to college almost five hours away from home was finding a local doctor near my campus. Having a physician close to where you live for the majority of the calendar year is a good idea regardless of your health situation, especially for people with T1D who require a little more health care than the average Joe or Jane.

If anything, your doctor near your school will serve as a safety net in case you need immediate care for something and cannot venture all the way home to your regular doctor. During my sophomore year of college, I suffered from a really bad case of migraines. I was in my bed for four to six hours almost every day for over a month. As a result of the migraines and irregular eating patterns, I started to lose control of my blood sugar levels. I talked with my parents on the phone, but there was not much they could do for me. Likewise, I went to see health services several times, but they were not specialists, either. My saving grace came when I started seeing a physician near my school. She prescribed me antimigraine medication to help me until I could make an appointment with a specialist, and also helped me establish basic routines to follow to stabilize my blood sugar. If I had never gone to see her, I do not know how I would have survived that semester.

Choosing to find a doctor near your school is totally up to you. Some people feel confident with just communicating closely with the doctors they have at home, while others prefer to have access to professional medical help closer to campus. If you decide to look for either a physician or an endocrinologist near your campus, the first people I would ask are your current doctors. They have colleagues all over the country, and on many occasions they will be able to point you in the right direction of a reliable doctor. Additionally, if you know any people living in the area where you go to college, ask if they recommend doctors in the area. The doctor that helped me with my migraines was referred to me by some close family friends who live close to my college.

ORDERING PRESCRIPTIONS

Most of what we have talked about thus far in this chapter is prevention based. This next topic, however, is directed toward your actual T1D care: ordering prescriptions. Personally, I did not order prescriptions myself when I lived at home; I would inform my parents I needed a prescription and they would order it for me. Looking back, it was something I could have done on my own. When I got to college, I soon found out that I needed to do it myself.

As an initial preventative measure, so you are always aware of when a prescription needs to be refilled, label the second-to-last box of all your supplies with a reminder that you are running low and need to order more soon. You can write this reminder on a sticky note, but I find it more effective to write it either on a piece of tape or directly on the box so it does not fall off.

In all honesty, it was surprisingly easy to learn how to order prescriptions. Even if you do not know how to order prescriptions, you should be aware of where you get them: pharmacies at CVS, Stop & Shop, Rite Aid, Walgreens, and so on. Check on the Internet or ask your health services office about the closest pharmacies to campus, and check to see which pharmacies are covered by your insurance by looking online or calling a number on your insurance card and talking with a representative from the insurance company.

Back home, I got my T1D prescriptions from Stop & Shop. Unfortunately, there are no Stop & Shops in the Burlington, Vermont, area, so I had to find a different pharmacy. I went to the closest CVS and had a conversation with one of the pharmacists behind the counter. I explained my situation to him, and he told me that if CVS was covered under my insurance, they would be able to transfer my prescriptions from the Stop & Shop pharmacy back home to the CVS pharmacy up in Vermont. I gave him my insurance card and ID, and within ten minutes, he had all my prescriptions on his computer. Ever since then, I have had absolutely no trouble ordering and filling prescriptions.

If you run out of a prescription, just go to the pharmacy and tell them you want a particular prescription refilled. They will be able to refill your prescription, but will most likely tell you to either wait around or come back in an hour or so, as it takes time to process

your request. Ordering your prescriptions by phone and then pick-
ing them up at your convenience saves you tons of time. To refill a
prescription by phone, call your pharmacy, at which point you will
have two options to choose from:

1. Go through the automated message and wait until you
   can select the option to refill a prescription. They usually
   have you either say the prescription number (Rx number)
   or type it in. The prescription's Rx number should be on
   the prescription paper you get every time you get the prescription filled.
2. Go through the automated message until you reach an actual
   pharmacist, and then just tell that person you want to refill a
   prescription. I prefer doing it this way because I find it more
   reassuring to talk to an actual human being.

One of the big troubles I faced during freshman year was finding
a ride to the pharmacy. Again, you have a couple of options. First,
you can learn the public transportation system around your college
and map out a way to get to and from your pharmacy. The public
bus system in Burlington, Vermont, is fairly reliable, and I used it
on several occasions. The other option is to find an upperclassman
who can either drive you to the pharmacy or let you borrow his or
her car. It might take a month or two to meet someone who has a car
and who feels comfortable helping you, but if this option presents
itself, take advantage of it. It gives you more flexibility and security
than public transportation, since many public transportation systems
have a strict time schedule and are usually filled with strangers.

SPORTS AND SOCIAL LIFE

The last few sections are simply reiterations of topics I have already
covered in previous chapters. I will briefly explain each topic and
some ways you can manage it with your T1D, and will also refer you
to the sections in this book that can help you further on these topics.

For more details on managing physical activity with T1D—in general and with respect to specific sports—see chapter 9, "Here's the Game Plan—T1D and Sports." If you are playing a sport in college, that means you are pretty good at your sport, so congratulations. Part of the reason for your success has probably come from your ability to correctly manage your blood sugar levels while playing that sport. Having said that, be aware of pushing your body too much if you do play a college sport. College athletics is a whole new ballgame compared to high school athletics. The intensity is kicked up about a thousand notches and the breaks are minimal. I have friends who play on sports teams in colleges who practice three times a day in the off-season! Know your body and know your limits. I understand that you have to put 100 percent into every practice or you will fall behind the rest of your teammates, but you will also fall behind if you have to sit out for an entire practice because you cannot control your blood sugar.

For more details on managing partying and drinking with T1D, see chapter 11, "Sex, Drugs, and Rock 'n' Roll." As I have mentioned before, you don't have to drink or party at college if you don't want to. It is simply a personal choice, and there are plenty of other fun things you can do that do not involve drinking and partying. However, if you decide you want to, be aware that college parties can happen multiple times every weekend and are probably ten times bigger than whatever you experienced in high school. Your legendary parties in high school are average parties at college. If you like partying, this can be exciting and fun, but it can also be dangerous. Similar to every other instance I have discussed in this book, know your limits and stay aware. Before you go out, put a snack on your pillow so you are more likely to remember to eat something before going to bed. Stay away from the jungle juice and do not drink anything whose origins and contents you do not know. There will be crowds of people at these parties, and 99 percent of them will not know you have T1D, so do not assume they do. Stick with your friends, and implement the guidelines I set out in chapter 11.

COLLEGE AND T1D—NO WORRIES

As I mentioned at the beginning of this chapter, do not stress and freak out that T1D is going to make college impossible. It doesn't have to. You are more prepared than you think you are. You have been preparing for this kind of freedom and independence for many years now. Remember that you were the one who made it through those tough first few weeks after your diagnosis. You were the one who learned how to count carbs, give yourself injections, and test for DKA (ketones). You have been managing your T1D for some time now. College is just another stepping-stone in your life where you can demonstrate to others and yourself that you are learning more and more how to take care of yourself and how to do it completely on your own. You will still make mistakes, and that is okay. Everyone makes mistakes. But just know that when you do go off to college, you *are* prepared to face the world with T1D at your side. Do not let it drag you down, but do not forget about it either. Have confidence in yourself, and do not hesitate to reach out and ask for help.

13

GETTING INVOLVED IN YOUR T1D COMMUNITY

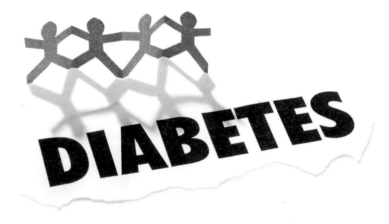

Congratulations! If you have made it to this chapter of my book, you have probably read the previous chapters and now know everything I know about T1D. As I have said many times before, realize that everything you have read in this book comes from experience; what

I have shared about T1D comes from my own life, as well as from the lives of family and friends who also have T1D.

Throughout the years I have had T1D, I have encountered my fair share of difficulties. In reflecting, I can seldom find a time when I was struggling and did not have someone, many times a fellow person with T1D, to lean on. Whether it was a doctor, teammate, cousin, or friend, all of the people with T1D I have known have gone out of their way to make sure I was okay. This mindset is not unique within the T1D community. People understand how hard this lifestyle can be at times, especially as a teen or young adult when so many things are changing in and outside your body. Those with T1D who have gone through the many struggles during their teen years may feel it is their duty to help others who are in the same boat as them. Obviously, they should not feel responsible for someone else's challenges—but many will want to do what they can to help, and that is reassuring.

When I started getting a grip on my own T1D management, I felt compelled to help others who were experiencing the same thing. But I did not know where to start. *Who should I talk to? How do I get involved? How can I make a difference?* If you want to get involved but are having these questions, this chapter may help you. Here, I will describe how I got involved in my T1D community and how you can too.

TALK WITH YOUR DOCTORS

A great starting place to get involved in your T1D community is to talk with your diabetes doctor. Sometimes your doctors know about certain mentoring programs or volunteer positions you can take advantage of. My diabetes doctor put me in contact with another doctor, Dr. Jodie, the psychologist on the team who hosted an "off to college day" for high school seniors with T1D. I was invited to serve on a college student panel and answered questions posed by both high school students with T1D and their parents. It was great being able to be a resource to people with T1D who were entering uncharted waters, waters I had already navigated.

I told Jodie I really enjoyed assisting on the panel and that I would be more than happy to get involved in any other related activities she knew about. A month or two later, Jodie invited me to take part in a mentoring program in which both she and I would sit with younger adolescent patients with T1D just to talk and eat snacks. I jumped on board immediately; I always enjoy talking with other people who have T1D. I was able to shed some light on subjects the kids were not too familiar with, and likewise, they taught me a few things too. I had never used a continuous glucose monitor (CGM) before, and several kids at the meeting were able to tell me what they thought about it (they all said they loved it). I find it incredible that even after being diagnosed with T1D over nine years ago, I can still learn new things about T1D and how to manage it. Since making contact with Jodie, I have worked with her at several additional T1D retreats and have met some wonderful people in the process.

JOIN/START A CLUB

Another way to get involved and help others with T1D is to join or start some kind of club. You can start one anywhere: in your town, at your school, or anywhere else where you will find people with T1D. It does not have to be a huge time or money commitment, either. The foundation of any T1D-related club or group should be to provide a safe haven where people with T1D can get the help they deserve. This foundation can be laid without millions of dollars and thousands of hours. In fact, I have noticed that the clubs

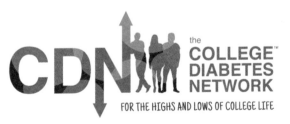

College Diabetes Network (CDN). Used with permission from Sarah Twomey-Mercurio.

with the most success are the ones that focus more on support and harmony and less on money.

Besides putting me into contact with Jodie, my diabetes doctor also told me to look into an organization called the College Diabetes Network (CDN) to get involved in the T1D community. It is a national organization that looks to create and support chapters of itself on college campuses across the nation. At the time, the organization already had over a hundred chapters in colleges nationwide! I looked them up on their website and was pleasantly surprised to learn that their goals and stances lined up almost exactly with my own; they wanted to provide an organization for people with T1D on college campuses who might need a support system and outlet.

I searched to see if there was a chapter at my school that I could join, but there was not. I contacted one of the directors of the CDN and asked if it was possible for me to start a chapter at my school. She was thrilled to hear that I wished to start a chapter and was instrumental in getting the CDN chapter at Saint Michael's College up and running. Since starting the chapter in the fall of 2016, we have participated in several community and volunteer events on campus and have plans to begin independently fundraising and volunteering soon. Additionally, we have reached out and met with the CDN chapter at the University of Vermont and are planning to participate in and host several events with them in the near future.

Participating in the CDN has done so much more for me than I ever could have imagined. The summer before my senior year of college, the CDN hosted a week-long retreat in Maine for some chapter members across the country. The retreat was one of the most eye-opening experiences of my life. I was introduced to other students and professionals from all over the country who felt the same way I did about helping others with T1D. Over the course of the week, I became friends with fellow chapter members, as well as individuals who worked for the CDN, whom I hope to remain friends with for the rest of my life.

MAKING CONNECTIONS: NETWORKING

My dad always told me, "It's not about what you know, it's about who you know." Over the years, I have concluded that his phrase holds some real truth. No matter what college you want to go to, job you want to land when you grow up, or place you eventually want to live, knowing someone who is already in that field can help you dramatically. People with T1D look out for their own, and by creating a club that helps other people with T1D or volunteering to help younger children with T1D, you are setting yourself up to meet people who could one day help you.

This might seem to be a rather selfish motive for doing something, but I am not trying to tell you that you should do these things out of self-interest. In fact, this selfish mindset does not even enter the minds of most people with T1D who are engaging in these sorts of community-based activities. All I am trying to say is that by integrating yourself into the T1D community, whether it is by being a panelist or mentor for younger people with T1D or starting a T1D outreach club in your town, you are actively helping the people around you, and that does not go unnoticed.

The summer before my senior year of college, I was contacted by a woman who had organized a fundraiser walk for T1D in Boston. She found my contact information from the CDN website, saw that I was the president of the CDN chapter at Saint Michael's College, and reached out to see if we would be interested in participating. These are the connections I want to emphasize. Putting yourself out there to help others with T1D can only help you in the future by opening doors and new avenues.

The T1D community is pretty tightly knit. People with T1D want to help each other because we understand the hardships the rest of the world does not. You are forced at a young age to become more responsible, organized, and mature. You have to test your blood sugar, administer injections, and worry about basically everything you eat and drink. Sometimes, it can be difficult and a downright pain in the ass. On several occasions, I have locked myself in my room and just cried about the fact that this is happening to me. *It's not fair. I didn't ask for this.* We know that; all of us in the T1D community know that. Sooner or later that mindset fades away, but the memory of it never does. People in the T1D community remember that feeling of helplessness and want to help anyone who is currently feeling what we felt when we were younger. In wrapping up this book, I will leave you with two things to think about that you should try to apply throughout your life as a person with T1D:

1. If you are feeling down on yourself for some reason, ask for help. Maybe you cannot get your blood sugar under control, or you do not like the new insulin system you are on, or you just need someone to vent to about everything that is going on in your life. The common term for this is called "diabetes burnout," and it happens to everyone. Reach out for help. Every person with T1D has felt these lows, and we want to help you desperately.

2. When you reach the point in your life when you feel you have a good handle on your T1D, get involved and help others who are facing the same struggles you did when you were younger. No one is asking you to cure T1D (we will let the scientists take care of that). But even if you just take some time to help a younger kid you know who was recently diagnosed, you will be helping the T1D community more than you know. Be the high to someone else's low.

We are all in this together and could all use each other's help in order to get through both the highs and lows of this roller-coaster of a lifestyle change.

GLOSSARY

Artificial pancreas: a hybrid closed-loop system; an insulin pump and continuous glucose monitor (CGM) that communicate with each other to independently and continuously check blood sugar levels and then modify basal insulin dosages based on those blood sugar readings.

Autoimmune disease: a disease in which the body's autoimmune system attacks parts of the body. In the case of T1D, your body attacks and kills your β-cells in your pancreas, which are responsible for producing insulin.

β-cells: the cells in the pancreas that produce insulin. These cells are damaged beyond repair in people with T1D.

Basal rate: a specific and steady amount of insulin that is received from an insulin pump to maintain normal blood sugar levels. This amount of insulin replaces longer-acting insulins taken with a daily injections regimen (Levemir or Lantus).

Bolus: a term used to describe a large amount of insulin given at one time. Bolus is commonly used to describe the amount of insulin you give yourself before a big meal, such as breakfast, lunch, or dinner.

Calories: the amount of energy contained within a food. As an example, if you look at a nutritional facts label on the side of an Oreo box and it reads, "Calories: 160," and the serving size is "3 cookies," this means that three Oreo cookies will be transformed into 160 calories of energy by the body.

Cannula: a part of an insulin pump that consists of a little plastic tube that connects the infusion site to the insulin reservoir in the pump.

Carbohydrates (carbs): a general term encompassing all the different kinds of sugars people eat. The body breaks down carbs into glucose molecules, which can then be used by your body to create energy. Under the carb umbrella are sugars, starches, and fiber.

Complex carbs (slow carbs): carbs that have a more complex molecular structure and therefore take more time for the body to break down. Examples of complex carbs are pasta, bread, potatoes, and whole milk.

Continuous Glucose Monitor (CGM): a device that independently and continuously tests blood sugar levels. CGMs are very helpful because they allow you to see trends in your blood sugar levels, which can help you make informed decisions with respect to correcting low and high blood sugar episodes.

Correction factor ratio: the ratio that indicates how much insulin is needed to correct a high blood sugar. As an example, if your correction factor ratio tells you to take one unit of insulin for every 30mg/dL your blood sugar is above 150, and you are 323, then you have to take seven units of insulin to correct that high blood sugar. (Here is how this insulin dose was calculated: you include all 30mg/dL units between 150 and 330. There are seven: 150, 180, 210, 240, 270, 300, 330.)

Daily injections: a type of insulin regimen for people with T1D that involves multiple injections every day. There are several different daily injection insulin regimens, which can vary based on types of insulins used and times of the day that require injections. This is the most common regimen for people who have been newly diagnosed with T1D because it allows your doctors to determine how your body responds to insulin and carbs.

Diabetes: a disease in which the body is not able to process sugar correctly and turn it into energy.

Diabetes burnout: a term used to describe the feeling of annoyance and dismay with T1D and all of its challenges, which results in the neglect of correct T1D management.

Endocrinologist: a physician who specializes in hormone disorders (insulin is a hormone). In this book, I commonly refer to endocrinologists as "diabetes doctors."

Fiber: a type of carbohydrate that comes from plants and is indigestible to humans. Since the body does not break down fiber, as a person with T1D who counts carbs, you can actually subtract some of the grams of fiber from the overall grams of carbs in the foods you eat.

Genes: the information coded in DNA. DNA is the body's "cookbook," which contains all the recipes to make what the body needs to survive. In the case of T1D, some of the genes may contain the wrong information, which ultimately causes the body to stop producing insulin.

Glucagon: a hormone produced by the pancreas that tells the body to release sugar stored in your cells so that it can be turned into energy. This is the main ingredient in emergency glucagon kits, which are used to treat extremely low blood sugar levels.

HbA1C: a measurement that is defined as the amount of sugar that is covering your red blood cells (measured in percentage). This is a common test your diabetes doctor will run on you every time you have an appointment, and is a good indication of your T1D management over the last three months. People with T1D want to have an HbA1C level under 7.0.

Honeymoon phase: the time in your life immediately following your T1D diagnosis. During this time, your body continues to produce a little insulin on top of what you inject yourself with. The duration and intensity of honeymoon phases varies greatly from person to person.

Hybrid closed-loop system: see **artificial pancreas.**

Hyperglycemia: high blood sugar; when the body does not have enough insulin, which results in too much free sugar floating around in the body. This excess sugar is mainly found in the blood and urine.

Hypoglycemia: low blood sugar; when the body does not have enough sugar to turn into energy to function properly.

Infusion catheter: the part of an insulin pump that is injected under the skin and that administers insulin into the body.

Insulin: a molecular key; a hormone produced by β-cells in the pancreas that "opens" the cells, allowing sugar to enter for conversion into energy.

Insulin pump: a device that contains fast-acting insulin and is used as an alternative insulin injection method to the daily injections regimen. There are many different types of insulin pumps with different features.

Insulin-to-carb ratio (I:C): the ratio describing the number of carbs you can eat for every 1 unit of insulin. For preteens it can be as much as 20 grams of carb for every 1 unit of insulin; whereas in adolescents the insulin-to-carb ratio is usually 1 unit of insulin for every 10 grams of carbs (or even less).

Diabetic Ketoacidosis (DKA): the process by which the body produces ketones. This occurs in people with T1D who have high blood sugar levels for an extended time.

Ketones: molecules that are produced when the body uses stored fat for energy. Ketones are commonly made when people with T1D need something to turn into energy but are unable to use sugar because of a lack of insulin.

Lancet: a finger pricker. People with T1D use this to get blood to test their blood sugar levels.

Pancreas: an organ in the human body that produces insulin and glycogen.

Pump: the mini-computer part of the insulin pump that regulates insulin delivery. Specific features of the pump vary by brand.

Simple carbs (fast carbs): carbs that primarily contain sugar. The body can break down simple carbs into glucose very easily, which means that they generally get into your system quickly. Examples of simple carbs are juice, fruit, candy, and syrup.

Sugar: a type of carbohydrate. Foods and drinks with a multitude of sugar are usually very sweet (candy, syrup, soda, etc.).

THC (tetrahydrocannabinol): the main chemical in marijuana. THC is responsible for marijuana's psychological effects.

Type 1 diabetes (T1D): a type of diabetes in which the body stops producing insulin. The body's autoimmune system attacks and kills the β-cells of the pancreas, which are responsible for producing insulin. T1D is a result of both the genes and the environment. People with T1D require daily doses of artificial insulin.

Type 2 diabetes (T2D): a type of diabetes that is mainly a result of poor diet and/or age. When too much stress is put on the pancreas, it stops responding to chemical signals and the body becomes resistant to the insulin. The body views its insulin as the "wrong key," and the cells cannot be unlocked. T2D can be controlled with oral medication and a good diet and exercise, although some people with T2D require daily doses of artificial insulin.

ACKNOWLEDGMENTS

I would like to thank Skyhorse Publishing, especially Katherine Mennone, for providing me with this amazing opportunity and helping me throughout the entire editing and publishing process; and my editor, Kim Lim, for her honesty and perseverance to be able to bring this book to a presentable form. Along the same lines, I would like to thank Dr. Tamborlane, Dr. Weinzimer, Dr. Jodie, and the rest of the Yale Pediatric Diabetes Team for providing professional expertise to help me further edit and correct the contents of the manuscript.

I would also like to thank Saint Michael's College for their continued help and support throughout this process. A special thanks to my advisor, Dagan Loisel; biology department chair, Declan McCabe; honors program director, James Byrne; and philosophy professor, Nicholas Kahm. Most importantly, a lifetime of thanks to my biology professor, Donna Bozzone, for meeting with me countless times to edit and revise the manuscript, and providing me with sound and experienced advice on issues concentrated both inside and outside the pages of the book.

And lastly, thank you to all my friends and family who have unconditionally supported me throughout this process. This dream never would have become a reality had it not been for all the love and encouragement I received. A special thanks to my mother, Nancy, father, Michael, and sister, Megan, for being the silent yet all-listening ears during both the highs and lows of this process.

INDEX